'An understanding of the complexity and of the creative and destructive power of the group lies at the heart of group analytic therapy and supervision. Whilst the setting and the boundaries of groupwork tend to remain relatively unchanged, the content and the outcome of practice is often surprising, often unexpected and arguably always new and different, emerging as it does from each new group. This book, the second in a series of three, brings that newness into clear focus. Thirteen writers provide a wealth of experience, knowledge and expertise. The reader is offered a kaleidoscopic view of current thinking and practice which is up to date, of the moment. The fifteen chapters are usefully grouped into four sections: Unconscious Processes, Working with Difference, Training Issues and Professional Issues. The lens through which the work of group supervision is viewed is specific to particular settings or areas of interest; the focus of the writing ranges from vivid vignettes of clinical practice to sophisticated and clearly argued theoretical positions. The multiple perspectives offered provide the reader with a wide-ranging view of analytic group supervision which will surely aid anyone involved in or thinking about being involved the demanding and ultimately highly rewarding task of working as a supervisor of a group.'

Leonie Hilliard, *Group Analyst, Training Group Analyst and Director of the Group Analytic Supervision Training at the Institute of Group Analysis, London*

'When I read this book, it seemed to me that built in to its culture, indeed in its very warp, is the sense of curiosity, mutuality, and reciprocity; for this to be the aim for the supervisor, for those seeking supervision, and for the "group as a whole". Each chapter has its own unique culture, and together they chart ways to openness. They make it safe to say the shameful. The supervision group takes place in the liminal space; where members can stay with moments of not knowing; analysing and accepting negative transference, ruptures and stuck-ness; and addressing the "anti-group". The book offered me space to think about and help solve long held riddles from my own early groups, family, training and own therapy. After reading this book, I believe I'm more confident, and competent, to help create a culture, in my present groups, that embraces other members own unique and diverse cultures; colonialism and ethnicity, holding in mind psychotherapy's western heritage. Reading this book also encourages me to rise to the challenge, post Covid, of working both in person and online.'

Roger Lloyd, *Chair of British Association of Psychoanalytic and Psychodynamic Supervision (BAPPS)*

Group Supervision and the Influence of Culture

Group Supervision and the Influence of Culture explores key themes in group analytic supervision, highlighting the value of thinking that encompasses different perspectives.

In this book, experienced group supervisors draw on their professional experiences from working with trauma, cross-cultural supervision, racism and shame. Part 1 explores unconscious processes, Part 2 looks at working with difference and Part 3 covers the training of supervisors of groups. Part 4 focuses on managing endings and learning from research how to maximise the benefits of group supervision. Finally, Part 5 explores ethics from a relational perspective, recognising that supervisory ethical practice is influenced by the culture of the day.

Group Supervision and the Influence of Culture will be essential reading for anyone providing group supervision, particularly therapists, counsellors, therapists, social workers, probation officers and healthcare staff who provide or receive group supervision. It will be an essential reference for trainees in group analytic supervision.

Margaret Smith is a retired psychodynamic psychotherapist and group analyst working in private practice with a special interest in group supervision. She was an independent member of the United Kingdom Council for Psychotherapy (UKCP), a Member of the Institute of Group Analysis (IGA) and British Association for Psychoanalytic and Psychodynamic Supervision (BAPPS) until 2023.

Group Supervision and the Influence of Culture

Edited by
Margaret Smith

Routledge
Taylor & Francis Group

LONDON AND NEW YORK

Designed cover image: 'Strawberry Moon', L.A. Simmons (2025)

First published 2026
by Routledge
4 Park Square, Milton Park, Abingdon, Oxon OX14 4RN

and by Routledge
605 Third Avenue, New York, NY 10158

Routledge is an imprint of the Taylor & Francis Group, an informa business

British Library Cataloguing-in-Publication Data
A catalogue record for this book is available from the British Library

Library of Congress Cataloging-in-Publication Data
Names: Smith, Margaret (Psychotherapist) editor
Title: Group supervision and the influence of culture / edited by Margaret Smith.
Description: Abingdon, Oxon ; New York, NY : Routledge, 2026. | Includes bibliographical references and index. |
Identifiers: LCCN 2025016901 (print) | LCCN 2025016902 (ebook) | ISBN 9781032719078 hardback | ISBN 9781032719054 paperback | ISBN 9781032719085 ebook
Subjects: LCSH: Group psychoanalysis | Psychoanalysts–Supervision of
Classification: LCC RC510 .G764 2026 (print) | LCC RC510 (ebook) | LC record available at https://lccn.loc.gov/2025016901
LC ebook record available at https://lccn.loc.gov/2025016902

ISBN: 978-1-032-71907-8 (hbk)
ISBN: 978-1-032-71905-4 (pbk)
ISBN: 978-1-032-71908-5 (ebk)

DOI: 10.4324/9781032719085

Typeset in Times New Roman
by Taylor & Francis Books

Contents

Acknowledgements

This book has been written by a team of supervisors who are enthusiastic about the benefits of providing group analytic supervision. Thank you to each of you for contributing your time and energy (unpaid) to produce this textbook. Your writing will be available to therapists providing group supervision in the future.

I would particularly like to thank Lee A. Simmons for the use of her artwork *Strawberry Moon* for the front cover of this book.

On a more personal note, I would like to thank all those who have provided me with both dyadic and group supervision through my working life, and thank you to the members of the supervision groups I have had the privilege to be a part of. There is so much wisdom to be gained from a well-functioning supervision group.

Thank you also to the Routledge team for your support in completing this book.

Margaret Smith

Contributors

Howard Edmunds is a training group analyst with the Institute of Group Analysis. He is qualified to provide group therapy for trainee group psychotherapists, offering both once and twice weekly group psychotherapy and individual psychoanalytic psychotherapy. Howard provides clinical supervision to individuals and organisations and clinical supervisor. As a member of the Institute of Group Analysis he has taught on the IGA Qualifying Course, IGA Foundation Course and IGA Diploma in Group Supervision. He has over 30 years' experience in a range of settings, including therapeutic communities, prisons, medium secure hospitals, NHS out-patient services and the voluntary sector. He is co-founder of Brighton Therapy Centre, a registered charity with a private practice in East Sussex.

Margaret Gallop is a group analytic psychotherapist in private practice with a special interest in supervision. She is a former co-convenor of the IGA Diploma in Supervision. She sees individuals and offers training and supervision in groups. She also co-convened the IGA Diploma in Supervision training.

Patrick Gannon is a group analyst, psychotherapist and supervisor, working privately in central London. He runs once weekly group analytic groups with patients who present with a variety of psychiatric conditions. He is also a supervisor, providing individual and group supervision to trainees at the Institute of Group Analysis and Manor House Centre for Psychotherapy and Counselling. In his role as clinical lead at Change of Harley Street, London, Patrick enjoys convening a comprehensive clinical CPD programme, enabling the clinicians at Change to reflect together around the theory and practice of contemporary psychological advancements.

Marina Gaspodini is a group analyst working in the NHS and in private practice. She is a member of the Institute of Group Analysis and of the UK Council for Psychotherapy. Marina supervises on the IGA Qualifying Course and on the Supervision of Supervision Diploma at the Institute of Group Analysis.

Frances Griffiths is an experienced group analytic supervisor working in private practice. As the current chair of CPJA ethics committee, she stresses the need for a space to think about ethical dilemmas. She is a member of a long-term peer supervision group and has taught on the IGA supervision course over a number of years.

Dr Maddy Loat is a clinical psychologist, psychotherapist, group analyst and clinical supervisor based in London, UK. She spent many years working in the NHS before moving into private practice where she currently works with individuals, couples and groups. She is an IGA training group analyst and conducts a twice-weekly analytic group in Central London. She is a full clinical member of the Institute of Group Analysis, the United Kingdom Council for Psychotherapy, the Health and Care Professions Council, and an associate fellow and chartered member of the British Psychological Society.

Dr Aisling McMahon is a clinical psychologist, integrative psychotherapist, group analyst and clinical supervisor, and has worked in various mental health settings in Ireland over the past 30 years. She is an assistant professor in psychotherapy at Dublin City University, where she is chair of a Professional Diploma in Clinical Supervision. With Peter Hawkins, Aisling is co-author of *Supervision in the Helping Professions* (2020, 5th edition). Aisling's specialist teaching and research interests are clinical supervision and practitioner development from training to retirement, areas in which she publishes and presents regularly.

Amélie Noack is a training group analyst for the Institute of Group Analysis, London, and a Jungian analyst. She worked for many years in private practice, teaching and supervising in the UK and abroad, as well as running the IGA's London Qualifying and Foundation Courses and working as the honorary secretary of the EGATIN (European Group Analytic Training Institutes Network) committee. She now works on the group analytic training course in GRAS, Germany, combining Jungian analysis, group analysis and Winnicott's contribution.

Fiona Pope is an experienced counsellor, supervisor and trainer. She currently supervises groups of trainee and qualified volunteer counsellors in a hospice setting where counselling is provided to patients with a terminal illness, their families and the bereaved.

Elisabeth Rohr, PhD, was professor for intercultural education at the University of Marburg, Germany, until 2013. Since her graduation as a group analyst in 1986, she has been working as a group analyst, supervisor, trainer and consultant in national and international, profit and non-profit organisations. In 2000, she managed to establish a group analytic training within a peace and reconciliation programme of the German government, trying to stabilise a traumatised society in Guatemala. Since then, she has worked in Palestine, online in Kenya, in El Salvador, Honduras and Guatemala, the UK and Denmark. She offers supervision in English, Spanish and German.

Lee Simmons is an art psychotherapist, EMDR consultant, integrative psychotherapist and supervisor. She is experienced working with adults, children and adolescents. Her clinical work has included supporting people at risk of deportation, expert witness, team training and consultancy for organisations such as EMDR UK, the British Association of Art Therapists, the NHS, Doctors of the World, CARAS, Freedom from Torture, the Refugee Council, Goldsmiths University of the Arts, the Priory Group, London Borough of Sutton Housing and Health and Second Floor Studios and Arts.

Joanna Skowrońska is a training group analyst, supervisor and teacher of psychotherapy and supervision in the Warsaw Institute of Group Analysis training. She is a former chairperson of the training committee, responsible for the training of supervisors, a certified psychotherapist of the Polish Psychological Association, and a graduate of the training for supervisors, Using the Group as a Medium of Supervision, at the Institute of Group Analysis in London. She runs seminars for supervisor candidates of the Polish Psychiatric Association. Joanna is interested in the factors that shape relationships between people and the applicability of small analytic groups in different social contexts, including supervision.

Margaret Smith is a retired psychotherapist and group analyst. She has worked both in the NHS and in private practice. Her previous experience includes teaching for the Liverpool diploma in psychotherapy training and the Tavistock D10 MA (Consultation and the organisation: Psychoanalytic approaches). She also co-convened the IGA Diploma in Supervision training from 2009 to 2018.

Introduction

The context for this book

This book is the second of three books about group analytic supervision. The first book, by Smith and Gallop, *Group Analytic Supervision* (2023), was also published by Routledge. Its aim was to paint a picture of the background, theory and practice of group analysis as an introduction to those who are new to this approach. |It was also intended as a short reminder for experienced group analysts who may need to explain the way they work for the therapists whose work they supervise.

The first book is designed to be dipped into so that each chapter can be read alone. It moves on to introduce the reader to the background, theory and practice of some key aspects of group analytic supervision through the lens of culture. These include the clinical hexagon, a model for group analytic supervision; dynamic administration, the supervisors' ongoing management of the supervisory frame; the supervisory alliance in group supervision; and the vital importance of self-care for therapists because they need to be robust in order to take care of other's needs. It includes the voice of the therapists and their experience of group supervision, drawing on and opportunistic research project using a small number of therapists' associations about their experience.

The book then looks at some of the key elements of ongoing supervisory practice. First, working with parallel process. It describes the development of the concept and its use and abuse in dyadic supervision. It continues with a résumé of how it developed within group analytic supervision and suggests ways that parallel process can enhance supervisory practice within group analytic supervision. Second, group analytic supervision welcomes and embraces difference as a way of enlarging the dialogue within the supervision group. It applies this to group analytic practice. Finally, it looks at the use of a two-way mirror, a practice used in systemic therapy, which can help supervisors in training to think about the dynamic aspects of their work as they emerge within their supervisory practice.

The aim of this book

This book tries to take account of culture, the aspects of society that are inside everyone who has lived within it, much of which a person may not be aware. This draws on the writing of SH Foulkes, who shone a light on some of the ways that our culture shapes our personalities and the way culture varies across different societies. Each chapter contains within it aspects of the wider culture that permeates the supervision group, the foundation matrix and also the unique culture as it emerges within the supervision group itself. It is written with each chapter taking up a different focus, but so that the reader can dip into it, picking out the areas that are of relevance to their work.

Group analytic supervision differs from dyadic supervision where two people interact with each other, one as the supervisor and the other as the therapist, where the two of them think together about the therapist's work. Group supervision adds what SH Foulkes talks about as the observer position, where there are observers who can think and reflect on the group discourse in a way that does not happen with a couple. The rest of the book adds to the content of the previous book *Group Analytic Supervision* by focusing on three areas that can benefit from the attention of those who offer supervision in groups. These can help the reader get a sense of how supervision group processes can deepen and enlarge the range of thoughts, feelings and associations. First, chapters reflect on unconscious processes in group supervision. Second, chapters cover different ways of thinking about working with difference. The book covers aspects of training from the perspective of supervisor, trainer and student. Finally, it looks at a number of professional issues that are important for the supervision of groups. A more detailed summary follows in the synopsis below

Synopsis of this book

Part 1: 'Unconscious Processes in Group Supervision' looks at ways of recognising and working with unconscious processes in group supervision. Chapter 1: 'Perturbations, Glitches and Glimpses in Group Supervision' looks at ways the supervision group can recognise unconscious processes that are having an adverse impact, viewing them as perturbations. Chapter 2: 'Towards a Group Analytic Model of Supervision' and Chapter 3: 'Narcissistic Investment as an Anti-Group Phenomenon' delve into aspects of supervisory practice, including the stance of the supervisor in the supervision group matrix—the web of group communications—tuning in to unconscious processes through the use of reverie. Part 1 moves on to think about the supervisor's role in recognising the therapists' analytic superego and finding ways to reduce the experience of shame and exposure; and, of equal importance, the supervisor's task of exploring and containing their own analytic superego as it emerges in the supervision group through self-reflection and the use of peer supervision of their work. This section finishes with Chapter 4: 'Dreams and Supervision'. Freud encouraged their use in psychoanalysis as the royal road to the unconscious. This chapter reflects on the journey of one supervisor of groups to value their dreams about supervision as containing previously unconscious, but potentially valuable, insights into their supervisory work.

Part 2: 'Working with Difference in Group Supervision' explores some of the challenges of working with difference in group supervision. It begins with Chapter 5: 'Cross-Cultural Issues in Supervision', inviting us to bear in mind some of the ways that different cultural norms can derail the supervisory process when they are not understood. Chapter 5 and Chapter 6: 'Working with Differences in Mind' look at ways that these differences can benefit the supervision group process. The final chapter in this section, Chapter 7: 'EMDR and Art Psychotherapy Group Supervision', is an example of applied group analytic supervision. It provides a window onto the way it can be used to support art psychotherapists in their work with traumatised groups of patients.

Part 3: 'Training and Group Supervision' begins with Chapter 8: 'Warp and Weft' on the supervision of students in training as therapists and some of the challenges involved in balancing the teaching needed to help students to adapt to the tension between creating a supervision group culture of nurture and openness and the need to assess their capability. Chapter 9: 'Cultural Sensitivity and Training for Supervisors of Groups' develops this theme but makes it appropriate for experienced therapists who, themselves, have much to offer. The final chapter in this section, Chapter 10: 'The Supervision Group as a Liminal Space', is written by an experienced therapist who describes the learning journey she underwent during her time training as a supervisor of groups. It introduces the concept of liminality to help navigate the various 'rites of passage' inherent in training and in the wider matrix of therapeutic work beyond.

Part 4: Professional Issues in Group Supervision looks at some of the professional issues that arise for supervisors of groups. Chapter 11: 'Some Thoughts on Planned and Unplanned Endings' includes aspects of dynamic administration, theory and practice as they relate to endings in group supervision, emphasising the importance of managing endings in a way that help rather than hinder the future supervisory experiences of the members of the supervision group. Chapter 12: 'Informing and Vitalising Group Supervision Practice', which looks at research into group supervision, provides an overview of research into, first, dyadic supervision and, second, group supervision. It concludes with recommendations that emerge from this research for good practice for supervisors. Chapter 13: 'Using the Group as a Medium of Supervision' concludes the section by applying some group analytic theory to supervision practice. It stresses the importance of the social dimension of the supervision group and the related concepts of mutuality and interdependence as the processes that underpin effective work.

Part 5: 'Ethics and Group Supervision' begins with Chapter 14: 'Is Supervision Ethical?', which explores ethical issues as they relate to group supervision, highlighting some of the ways that our cultural lens shapes our ethical standards. The final chapter, Chapter 15: 'Group Supervision, Ethics and the Influence of Culture', continues by tracing the development of ethical practice from the eighth century BCE, the period when the first societies emerged, looking at some of the similarities and differences across cultures.

The title of this book

Our book title, *Group Supervision and the Influence of Culture*, has been chosen in recognition that group analytic supervision is, above all else, a relational and collaborative experience. SH Foulkes, the founder of group analysis, described the individuals within a group as being like nodes inside the network of the group. He recognised that individuals are not a closed system because they absorb their environment through the communications taking place in their group. This matrix encompasses many levels, from the wider society to the inner workings of the mind (Foulkes, 1964: 117, 290). This book captures some of the ways that culture shapes the work of the supervision group and how the supervisor of groups works with this.

The intended readership

This book was drawn from the experience of a range of experienced supervisors providing group supervision. It is intended for practitioners who are providing group supervision or are planning to do so. It will be of use to supervisors of groups working in different fields, including group analysis, counselling and psychotherapy, nursing, social work, probation, education, religious, music and drama therapy.

It holds in mind the influence of the surrounding culture, while also addressing some of the benefits and challenges of group analytic supervision. It was written to support supervisors of groups with helping their groups to recognise and work with unconscious processes. The section on working with difference gives examples from experts in the field about how they help the group use different perspectives to enhance the work of the group. It The chapters on training will be of particular relevance to institutes who offer postgraduate training for therapists in group analytic supervision, including the Institute of Group Analysis in London and also institutes across Europe, Australia and America. It will be of interest to training institutions who provide group supervision to their students and to charities who offer counselling and therapy services.

References

Foulkes SH (1964) *Therapeutic Group Analysis*. George Allen and Unwin.
Smith M and Gallop M (2023) *Group Analytic Supervision*. Routledge.

Part I

Unconscious Processes in Group Supervision

Chapter 1

Perturbations, Glitches and Glimpses in Group Supervision

Howard Edmunds

According to Collins Online Dictionary (2025) a perturbation is a 'small continuous deviation in the ... orbit of a planet or comet, due to the attraction of neighbouring planets'.

Introduction

How can supervisors and supervisees best understand the therapy relationship when the most significant processes are unconscious? Supervisors must decode communication that is both complex and encrypted. Complex because of the vast quantity and layering of information. Encrypted because what is most feared by supervisees and patients is often disguised or hidden from view. When trauma, vulnerabilities and shameful secrets are avoided, supervision gets stuck. It comes to resemble a talking shop or coffee morning and time is lost 'paddling in the shallows' (Behr and Hearst, 2005: 146). To reveal unconscious processes, we need to know *where* to look, how to safely *reveal* and how to *contain* the results. Perturbations, glitches and glimpses are metaphors for ruptures, tears and blocks in the supervision group's dialogue. They include the absence of a response, omissions and avoidances, repetition, and barely audible whispers. It is these distortions that alert us to the presence of hidden or unconscious processes. To understand how this works, we need to first explore the concept of parallel process.

Parallel process

Parallel process is ever-present in all supervisory relationships, but often goes unnoticed. It describes the way in which the supervisee-supervisor relationship mirrors the therapist-client relationship and vice versa. Searles first writes about the phenomenon whereby the supervisor's emotions could be 'a reflection of something which has been going on in the therapist-client relationship' (Searles, 1955: 136–137). Ekstein and Wallerstein observe two-way mirroring where the therapist-supervisor relationship also changes the client-therapist relationship (Ekstein and Wallerstein, 1958). They consider the therapists'

DOI: 10.4324/9781032719085-2

problems in learning in supervision as mirroring the client's defences to therapy. Caligor replaces the term parallel process with reciprocal process to further underline the two-way nature of the mirroring process (Caligor, 1984: 25–26). Ekstein and Wallerstein focus on situations where both supervisor and therapist get stuck because of strong emotions, such as rage or feeling useless. However, whilst the focus of Searles and Ekstein/Wallerstein is mainly on individual supervision, Caligor points out the advantage of using a supervision group or reflecting team. He demonstrates how a supervision group can offer multiple perspectives; how a group discussion gives the supervisor time to step back and examine the process; how the supervision group is itself a system that in turn acts as a mirror to the system of the client's internal world. The most commonly occurring example is where a client's resistance is mirrored in the supervision group; the supervisee is reluctant to talk about their work and feels at odds with the group. This is similar to one of the core insights of group analysis, which utilises the tendency of the therapy group to mirror and 'amplify' the internal dynamics of its members (Pines, 1995: 2). When I was taking part in the IGA supervision training, one of the seminar leaders referred to the supervision group as an echo chamber. Caligor alerts us as to the challenges of group supervision in provoking anxiety and defences. The clinical vignettes that follow illustrate parallel process working in both directions.

Perturbations

The *Encarta Dictionary* defines perturbation as both noun and verb. As a noun: 'a disturbed and troubled state'. As a verb: 'the act of disturbing and troubling somebody'. This captures the dual nature of perturbation in supervision where a supervisee arrives unsettled and is also unsettling to the group. The supervisor feels as if something is up but does not understand what is going on as the cause remains hidden. The third definition of perturbation is from astronomy: 'A deviation in an astronomical object's orbit or path caused by the gravitational attraction of another astronomical object'. In supervision, the client, therapist, organisation and supervision group are like planets or solar systems interacting: each causing perturbations in the others' orbits. I use the term perturbation in preference to 'enactments', because it captures the experience where something is missing, incongruous or not mentioned. This is in contrast with the term enactment which describes actions driven by unconscious impulses but which are easier to identify.

A perturbation is where a communication is not responded to: the absence of a *response* or *reply* to an event or communication. Its prototypes are ruptures in the early mirroring between carer and baby; failures that inevitably reappear in the therapy relationship due to their fundamental nature. The importance of a responsive supervisory relationship is as fundamental as the importance of early mirroring between infant and carer described by

Gerhardt (Gerhardt and Matthes, 2011). When mirroring breaks down the baby disengages or slumps. Perturbations are also created by psychic explosions: traumas. Traumas induce a freeze response as a defence against overwhelming emotions. A minor trauma evokes a momentary freeze while a major trauma can evoke a dorsal response, where communication and thinking are impossible. In supervision, perturbations are used as indicators. The absence of a call and a reply alerts us to the presence of hidden or unconscious processes and trauma.

Perturbations in the supervision relationship

Vignette I

A multidisciplinary supervision group meets in a mental health team working to support and contain severely disturbed clients living in Marseilles, a coastal city with high levels of crime and social deprivation. The group supervisor is initially greeted with enthusiasm by all the group members (Joseph, Aurélie and Françoise) who had been asking for more support with work stress for some time. However, one supervisee regularly arrives for the group 10 minutes late. Nobody comments or responds to this. The group supervisor is also mute—they reflect on the strange sense of dread that they are experiencing as they recognise that they need to address what is happening. At the start of the fifth week, the supervisor addresses the issue.

—SUPERVISOR: Françoise, I want to ask you about your lateness.
—FRANÇOISE: I have been. You're right. I'm sorry. I … [bursts into tears].
—AURÉLIE: It's OK, Françoise. You're OK. [Aurélie puts an arm around her.]
    Françoise continues to sob deeply.
—JOSEPH: [Joseph reaches over to Françoise] Come on. It's time to go.

The three other group members move to support Françoise, and as a group, lift her to her feet and walk her gently out of the room. The session ends. One group member comes back looking embarrassed—to apologise. She is too upset to talk this week, and we will have to resume the group next week. The supervisor experiences an overarching feeling of fear that they have caused harm.

Everyone can agree that it is good to reflect on our work—until someone touches a raw nerve. In this case, the size of the perturbation is proportionate to the magnitude of what has been repressed.

The next week, Françoise returns to the group. Her lateness told a story of burnout and fear after the recent death of a key client, Mrs D, by suicide. This followed the death by drowning of Mrs D's four-year-old daughter.

Françoise believed that she might have prevented the tragedy. She imagined colleagues and relatives partly blamed her. She dreaded the inquest and had been unable to write her report, which was becoming more and more urgent.

Holding a very high case load, as was true for all of the team at that time, she was working many hours of overtime to try to ensure that she was completely on top of all her other cases. This impossible task was putting her under a huge strain. Unknown to her colleagues and manager she was staying on hours after the usual working day, and then struggling in late for work the following morning, exhausted. As the group spoke about the tragedy of the parent and child it was possible to begin to face the sadness and powerlessness that the team felt and to start to discuss the wider problem of trying to support the most vulnerable clients with limited resources. An open verdict as to the cause of death of the child left unanswered questions as to how the child had come to drown.

The group's discussion of her client's death enabled Françoise to become curious about Mrs D's situation before her suicide. She was also more able to ask for help from her manager and went to the inquest. On her return she reported having found out lots of significant details of the case which helped her to begin to make some meaning from it. The atmosphere in the group had changed. Françoise had needed to hear from her colleagues that it was not her fault Mrs D had committed suicide. Françoise then disclosed that her four-year-old sister had drowned when she, Françoise, was a child.

Discussion

Although the lateness was an obvious problem for the group, the perturbation was the lack of response or reply to the lateness by group members. The supervisor reported a strong feeling of dread in raising it with Françoise. They had avoided it for several weeks but could not explain why. In raising it, the supervisor failed to recognise that they were perhaps the least well equipped to explore the problem. This leads to a different methodology of working with perturbations, covered in the section on managing shame further below.

Vignette 2. Perturbation as an absence

In an inner-city supervision group, Frank introduced the case of a client, Ali, who was in his 40s and still living with his mother. Ali spent most of his time playing computer war games; and he had once threatened his female care worker with a knife. As a young infant, Ali had been exposed to violence between his parents. In view of his risk, the group agreed with Frank's assessment that Ali needed continued monitoring and help to move to supported housing and to engage more in community activities. Two sessions later he was not mentioned in the group and, when asked, Frank reported that the consultant had decided to discharge Ali and the plan to move him to supported housing had been dropped. Frank said there was nothing more to say—the client was going to be taken off his caseload.

—SUPERVISOR: So, if I've got this right; you've been told that your care plan is to be dropped and you have not been given any idea of the consultant's thinking. What do you make of that?

—FRANK: [looks puzzled] I think it is to do with the pressure to discharge clients when we get so many referrals.

—SUPERVISOR: But it sounds like there has not been any discussion about that?

—FRANK: Welcome to our world!

At the next session, Frank reported that, having raised his concern, the decision had been reversed and he was now back on the case of finding Ali supported housing. However, he still did not have any idea about why the consultant had wanted to discharge Ali.

Discussion

The perturbation in the supervision group is the moment when Frank omits to bring an important update about Ali to the supervision group and has 'nothing more to say' on the matter. The perturbation in this case reveals the impact of trauma in the client, resource pressures in the organisation and power relations within the clinical team. The supervisor is alerted by a perturbation and provides the missing response to the chain of events.

Vignette 3: The supervisor as the trigger for the perturbation

Peter presented a session with a depressed and anxious client Carl who had missed a session after attending his sessions regularly for nine months. Carl could not come because of his partner's antenatal appointment. At this point, the supervisor commented that they felt foggy and cut-off while Peter had been talking and wondered what that might be about. Peter joked that he was probably boring the supervisor. He recalled that Carl had said how he was afraid that he was boring. This led to a new idea—was Carl worried that Peter was more interested in him as a new father rather than in him as a person?

Discussion

The perturbation of the supervisor's reflection on their own lack of emotional responsiveness to this client helped the supervisor to link this with the client's experience of feeling unimportant to others. In later sessions it emerged that Carl's mother expected him to give his younger brother his, Carl's, toys whenever the younger brother wanted them. Carl did not have a sense of having anything that was just for him. It emerged that he had a core belief that he would never be loved or valued for who he was.

Glitches

A glitch is an intermittent fault in a system that makes it difficult to troubleshoot. It can appear mysterious or seemingly inexplicable. Computer programmers are familiar with glitches—the program freezes or repeats the same message over and over, much to the frustration of the user.

A glitch in supervision is where the message also gets repeated or is overstated. For example, repetition might appear with a client who repeats over and over their story of abuse or neglect without emotion or ability to connect to others in the group on an emotional level. This gets repeated in the supervision relationship where boredom and disinterest creep in, so that the client gets overlooked. Overstated communication might be any of the following: too nice, too cold, too aggressive, too friendly, or too focused on the supervisor, group or individual.

Vignette 4: Being flooded

A supervision group of newly qualified counsellors in private practice meets weekly. A therapist presents a female client in great detail, relaying a verbatim account of each session in such a way that there is no time for discussion about the work. It emerges that this kind of flooding of the space is also how the client relates to the practitioner. The client needs to explain in great detail their problem, their analysis of the problem, and all the specific cultural and social factors that they are affected by. In the supervision group, the supervisor and other group members are similarly stymied. The supervisor shares that, despite being given all the information, they are finding it hard to think about what might be going on between the client and the therapist. The therapist responds with a huge sigh of relief. That is exactly what they are struggling with—they feel as if the client cannot allow them space to think and they are feeling increasingly inadequate.

Discussion

The therapist presented an overly detailed account of their work and invited the supervision group to be a passive witness without allowing them to offer their thoughts and reflections. This mirrors the therapy relationship. The client had forcefully excluded their therapist and appears to want to enlist them purely as a witness. This led to a glitch in the supervision group—a flooding of information. On noticing the glitch, the supervisor described their struggle to think. Which in turn enabled the therapist to talk about their own sense of inadequacy. In later sessions, the client started to talk about their sense of shame and inadequacy. They had been enlisting their therapist as a passive witness to defend against their deep sense of shame. Shame is explored more fully below.

Glimpses

Glimpses are brief or whispered communications that are easily missed: something important is briefly mentioned, a client is rarely discussed in supervision, or a shocking experience is described without affect. Glimpses are like icebergs—a small thing on the surface hide a large obstacle underneath. They are the result of high levels of ambivalence: a wish to be heard and a fear of the possible consequences. They are a kind of test—if you really want to hear me, you must move closer to hear what I am saying.

Vignette 5: Reflections on a boundary change

A trainee psychodynamic counsellor, Lucy, had agreed with a client, Sonia, that she change from weekly to fortnightly sessions. The trainee came to supervision and realised she had agreed to the fortnightly sessions without any discussion in her supervision group. The supervisor noticed that Lucy had not talked about her client Sonia for some time, having spoken about her a lot during her early sessions. They asked Lucy if she had a sense of what was stopping her talking about this client. Lucy shared an image she had of the supervisor stepping in and trying to control her work with this client, rather like a controlling mother. She then recalled Sonia's difficulty in separating from her mother and how Sonia had cut her hair and kept it secret from her mother until it was all done. Sonia had expected her mother to try to take over.

Discussion

The way that Lucy presented Sonia was such that we only glimpsed something that had already been done and had been hidden. But this leads to an understanding of how afraid the client is of being taken over by others. Lucy mirrors this fear by hiding her work from the supervisor.

Using perturbations, glitches and glimpses to encourage active participation and observation

One advantage of group supervision is the possibility of having both participants and observers. A practitioner presenting their work and another reacting and sharing their response provides high levels of participation. Those who are silent however, can be valuable observers. And with more people their multiple 'lines of sight' make it more likely that a perturbation will be spotted (Edmunds, 2017). Looking out for perturbations can resemble a kind of play or game, whereby it helps to keep everyone focused. However, perturbations, by definition, will always come as a surprise and often evoke shame responses, as was experienced by Françoise in Vignette 1. Supervisors who explain the value of concepts like perturbations and parallel process at the outset of supervision may reduce this risk.

Managing shame reactions in supervision

Supervisors or supervisees acting out of the ordinary or going off task often assume that they have a personal issue or deficiency. This gets in the way of being curious and they may hide or avoid their perturbation altogether. In Vignette 1, Françoise's reaction is extreme but not uncommon. It reflects the secondary trauma that she had witnessed.

Vignette 1: The supervisor returned to the previous session and wondered what it was that had made it so difficult to talk about Françoise's lateness. Françoise volunteered how she had felt 'shoddy' about her work for some time, and that the supervisor's drawing attention to her lateness had felt overwhelming. Everyone knew this but nobody was able to say it.

In Vignette 1, by asking Françoise about her lateness the supervisor asked the person who was least equipped to answer.

How might the supervisor have made use of the group's resources instead?

If the problem is considered in the context of the group, rather than just being seen as residing in one individual, the way forward is to repair the lack of reply. This suggests that rather than asking Françoise, the supervisor asks the whole group what is making it so hard for them to respond to Françoise's lateness; what stops them from asking her if she is OK. Groups are unique in their ability to process trauma in this way. This use of the group is described by the myth of Perseus and Medusa.

The supervision group as mirror

In acting as a mirror, the supervision group in Vignette 1 is able to act as a mirror for Mrs D and Françoise's shame. In the Greek myth of Perseus and Medusa, Perseus is given a mirror with which to look at Medusa without being turned to stone. Shame, death and suicide were Medusa's serpents and the supervision group was perturbed but not frozen. Like a shield, they could not reflect the trauma with its full force and were too many-sided to be completely taken over. When the inquest of Mrs D's suicide came and went without comment, the supervisor asked how it went. The group's perturbation was to avoid the topic and at this point it was the supervisor who remembered. But at another time, it could have been another group member who was able to step back and notice the perturbation. If one person goes blank, it is unlikely that all members of the supervision group will be paralysed at the same time. The supervision group works because all members need each other and are able to recognise this rather than deny it.

Conclusion

Perturbations, glitches and glimpses are indicators of unconscious conflicts. They tell us where to look. A perturbation is an absence of call and reply.

Vignettes 1–3 illustrate how this absence of responsiveness in a supervisory relationship can indicate the presence of trauma in the client or practitioner. Glitches, in contrast, are overstated communications, where flooding is used as a defence against shame. Glimpses, like whispers, are easily missed.

Supervision groups enable multiple roles for participants and observers. It is unusual for the whole of a supervision group to become frozen at the same time. When a whole supervision group is caught in a perturbation, before long, the supervisor or a supervisee will step back and wonder aloud what is going on. In observing their own process, the supervision group is more able to catch these moments and make full use of their implications. The supervision group thus acts as a mirror so that the original trauma, with all its shock waves, can be faced. Supervisors who disclose their own struggles to remain focused on the task, can free up the supervision group to be curious about these breaks and distortions in their own communication. However, when perturbations are noticed and examined, there is usually an explosion of repressed emotion and shame that is hard to contain. Repairing a breakdown of communication in the supervision group as a whole is more likely to succeed than putting all the focus on an individual supervisee. Rather like a treasure hunt, seeking out perturbations encourages play and curiosity. Repairing tears and ruptures in communication gets easier with practice, with the result that supervision groups find their own ways to manage shame and so remain curious about what they might uncover. As a parallel process, when a supervision group recovers its capacity to communicate and think creatively, these benefits are transferred to the therapy relationship and therefore to the client.

References

Behr H and Hearst L (2005) *Group-Analytic Psychotherapy: A Meeting of Minds.* Whurr Publishers.

Caligor L (1984) Parallel and Reciprocal Processes in Psychoanalytic Supervision. In: Caligor L, Bromberg PM and Meltzer JD (eds), *Clinical Perspectives on the Supervision of Psychoanalysis and Psychotherapy.* Springer, pp. 1–28.

Collins Online Dictionary (2025). https://www.collinsdictionary.com/.

Edmunds H (2017) Model for Reflective Practice and Structured Group Supervision. *Group Analytic Contexts.* Newsletter available at *Contexts*, pp. 72–81. https://groupa nalyticsociety.co.uk/wp-content/uploads/2018/12/C78-FINAL.pdf.

Ekstein R and Wallerstein RS (1958) *The Teaching and Learning of Psychotherapy.* Basic Books.

Gerhardt S and Matthes M (2011) *Why Love Matters: How Affection Shapes a Baby's Brain.* Routledge, pp. 80–97.

Pines M (1995) Introduction. In: Sharpe M (ed.), *The Third Eye: Supervision of Analytic Groups.* Routledge.

Searles HF (1955) The Informational Value of the Supervisor's Emotional Experiences. *Psychiatry*, 18 (2): 135–146.

Towards a Group Analytic Model of Supervision

The Matrix and Reverie in Group Supervision

Patrick Gannon

Introduction

In Chapter 2, I explore how the use of the particular conceptual framework of 'matrix and reverie' (Berman and Berger, 2007: 241) helped to contain a difficult dynamic that played out in my supervision group. First, I describe the group composition and culture, and our beginning sessions, demonstrating that each supervisee brought their own foundational culture to the 'dynamic matrix' (Foulkes, 1990: 213). I reference 'dynamic administration' (Behr and Hearst, 2005: 42–45) along with boundary setting and the important task of 'holding' (Winnicott, 1971: 166). Second, I show how the group began to develop its own dynamic culture through the 'supervision group process' (Plant and Smith, 2012), looking at 'parallel processes' (Searles 1955) between the patient work presented, the supervision group and my peer supervision group. To conclude, I demonstrate how the group began to make use of a 'reflecting team' approach (Smith and Plant, 2012; Smith, 2019), enabling the supervisees to feel more confident in their clinical practice, harnessing a culture of difference and democracy, in the service of the supervision group. I also reflect on my own development as a group supervisor. With the use of vignettes, I refer to one very particular patient presented and the associated group dynamic/culture, demonstrating how the therapist-patient work progressed in using the group as the medium for supervision.

Group composition and group culture

After interviewing a number of prospective supervisees for my new supervision group, I decided to begin with three experienced clinicians—a consultant psychiatrist (Andrew), a clinical psychologist (Elisa) and an integrative psychotherapist (Hannah). For the purposes of confidentiality, I have changed their names. At the time of advertising this new supervision group, the UK encountered a rapidly evolving cultural change as it entered the second lockdown due to the Covid-19 pandemic. As a result, these interviews were held online and, as it happened, the supervision group turned out to be an online

DOI: 10.4324/9781032719085-3

supervision group—so we all had to adapt to a way of working that we had never imagined previously. As the group members and I shared our anxieties about working online and the loss we all experienced around in-person working, I noticed a culture of openness and tolerance emerging in our communication with each other. The task of dynamic administration now included an open discussion around Zoom etiquette, boundaries in terms of a private and confidential space, an appropriate fee for the online group supervision, and the importance of giving notice to the group around absences. Noack asserts,

> Dynamic administration creates an immutable division and clear boundaries between inside and outside the group, which in turn provides within the group a secure space for psychic exploration. The group related focus on dynamic administration enables the supervisor to highlight the importance of the establishment of these basic aspects of therapeutic activity.
>
> (Noack, 2009: 7–8)

As I had previously set up private group analytic groups, this task of dynamic administration did not feel too onerous. However, the big difference in setting up this group was to do with the importance of the loss of face-to-face contact and something of what a disembodied experience of supervision would mean for each supervisee's clinical work and the formation of the group as a whole (Foulkes, 1964: 253). One advantage of this discussion was that we were immediately able to look at the parallel processes of online group dynamics and the supervisees' online clinical work. Such parallel processes were to emerge also between my online peer supervision group and this new group. I discuss these processes in more detail later. In setting up this new group, my peer supervision group played a crucial role in helping me shape the group culture in respect of advertising the group, deciding on the prospective members, setting the fee, date, and time of the group, the frequency of the group, and GDPR forms, etc.

Smith and Gallop assert,

> Supervision groups have their own culture, and their engagement shapes the group experience as they use the supervisory space for exploration of their responses to the therapy work ... the 'good enough' supervisors of groups provide a holding environment where the group can be genuine and honest and engage in serious and creative play revealing personal associations and experiences, phantasies and dreams.
>
> (Smith and Gallop, 2023: 107)

Of course, all groups have their own culture. Through the task of 'dynamic administration' (Behr and Hearst, 2005), I already had a sense of the differences and similarities in the training backgrounds of each supervisee, and I wondered how the 'cultural norms and values' (Foulkes 1990: 275) would play out in this supervision group.

The clinical hexagon and supervision group process

To my great relief, all three supervisees entered my Zoom waiting room on the agreed start date. Although I had known Andrew, Elisa and Hannah previously in a professional capacity, they did not know each other and so I invited them to introduce themselves to each other. All three clinicians are in private practice, experienced and successful. I also have much experience of private practice. I have over 25 years of working as a psychotherapist in both the National Health Service (NHS) and private practice. All three clinicians were analytically minded and yet each used different therapeutic approaches in their clinical practice, which I thought would contribute to rich and interesting discussions in the group. Elisa was also trained in dynamic interpersonal therapy (DIT), Hannah was also qualified as a life and business coach and Andrew had a qualification in cognitive analytical therapy (CAT). Dynamics of power, privilege and hierarchy immediately imbued the culture of the supervision group.

Within the first 30 minutes of our first supervision group the competition in the group was palpable. As each supervisee introduced themselves, in my countertransference, I could feel an immense pressure to say something intelligent and insightful. Mindful of my own need to be liked and validated by the group, I was conscious of the importance of not acting into my countertransference so that I might be able to hold the analytic stance of 'not knowing' (Bion 1962) both for me and for the group. Drawing on my own training in group analysis and on my training in group analytic supervision, I remembered a number of discussions on the usefulness of paying attention to the 'analytic frame' (Crawford, 2005: 60) as a way of holding the anxiety ever-present in the beginnings of any group. I was also holding in mind the usefulness of the 'clinical hexagon' (Smith and Gallop, 2023: 81) and the importance placed on the task of moving the group's communication process between the areas of dynamic administration, the therapy, the therapist, the supervision group dynamics, the supervisor's countertransference and the organisation. As Smith says,

> The clinical hexagon offers a compass for the supervisor who can use it to think about where to focus. It provides a framework to support the supervisor of groups to work with the multi-perspective contributions of group supervision.
>
> (Smith and Gallop, 2023)

Vignette 1

After each supervisee introduced themselves, I commented that I was struck by the similarities of their patient populations. The supervisees spoke about working in central London with high-functioning borderline personality disorder (BPD) patients, who were all referred privately. They each spoke about the challenges they faced with this patient group in terms of their patients' mood swings, intrusive thoughts, emotional dysregulation and their ever-present narcissistic need for wanting answers and wanting 'to be fixed'. Each supervisee admitted that they felt they disappointed their patients in *not* being able to fix them. I wondered with the group if perhaps a similar dynamic might play out in this new group where there would be pressure on me to provide answers and that they might feel disappointed with me or with each other. In this discussion, as all four of us resonated with the feeling of disappointment, I felt the group to be more at ease, and I certainly noticed myself relax a little. We ended this session by deciding on how we would allocate the time each week. We agreed that the first half hour would be a general check-in and then each supervisee would take it in turns to present one of their patients each week. Hannah said she felt relieved that she had a safe space to bring her clinical work where there would be the support of other colleagues.

In reporting back to my peer group the following week, I spoke about feeling relieved that my supervision group had begun. One of my peers wondered if the group had already idealised me as 'the expert', handing over their authority to me as the supervisor. I did not like hearing this but, as time progressed, I had to admit that I was idealised and what emerged in the group matrix (Foulkes, 1964), in the midst of the competition and rivalry, was something of an unconscious re-enactment of sibling rivalry, paralleling similar unconscious rivalries within the lives of the patients presented. Searles (1955) suggests that 'processes at work currently in the relationship between patient and therapist are often reflected in the relationship between therapist and supervisor' (Searles, 1995: 135). Searles believed that the emotion or reflection experienced by the supervisor was the same emotion felt by the therapist in the therapeutic relationship. It seemed to me that, even at this very early stage of group supervision, there were many parallel re-enactments between the patient work presented, my supervision group and my peer supervision group. I return to this later when discussing my peer supervision group.

The conceptual framework of the matrix and reverie in my supervision group

In speaking of the matrix and reverie in group supervision, Berman and Berger assert,

16   Group Supervision and the Influence of Culture

the whole experience brings the supervisee back from the emotional exile he is likely to be banished into when struggling with his professional difficulties on his own. It strengthens his ability to contain his patients' feelings and to develop some faith in his own resources.

(Berman and Berger, 2007: 245)

In thinking of the group as the medium of supervision, I was especially drawn to Berman and Berger who seek out a conceptual frame that, when applied to group supervision, allows for the development of a potential learning space for all its participants. They suggest that Bion's notion of reverie (Bion, 1962) and Foulkes' concept of the matrix (Foulkes, 1964), when bound together, can provide such an environment.

Bion describes reverie as a state of mind in which alpha functions allow for the experience of a dreamlike drifting into one's associations, feelings and loose personal musings. It enables a mother to feel her baby's emotional state and contain it. Her containing capacity is transformative for her infant and renders their feelings bearable and growth producing. Berman and Berger suggest that group supervision can be perceived as a process of generating meaningful thoughts and experiences for reverie (Berman and Berger, 2007: 241). These thoughts and experiences are *co-created* by all group members, including the supervisor. These personal, private aspects of a therapist's inner life, namely their reverie, constitutes a most valuable asset in the processing of therapeutic issues by a supervision group. Berman and Berger believe in the collective 'group reverie', which is co-created by the compiled personal associations (and associations to the initial associations) that members contribute in the process of sharing with each other the specific way in which the presented material resonates in their private world (Berman and Berger, 2007: 241).

Foulkes may have had something similar in mind when he referred to the 'group's chain of associations' as 'free floating discussion' or his view of the group as a 'network of associations'. He describes the matrix as 'the hypothetical web of communication and relationship in a given group' (Foulkes, 1964: 292). This notion of matrix emphasises that individual members in a group are part of a collective tapestry that creates a network of mutual associations and, at the same time, defines each individual in it. As such, the individuals in the supervision group can participate in an open discourse, generate a creative dialogue between group members, increasing each therapist's capacity to contain the emotional complexity of their patients. When the notion of reverie and the concept of matrix are bound together, the supervision group can become a containing place for supervisees to discuss and explore the challenges they face in their clinical work.

Vignette 2

As the weeks progressed, each supervisee presented a variety of patients, allowing for some very interesting and stimulating clinical discussion. During the fifth session Hannah presented Mary, a 35-year-old executive assistant working in a city bank. Mary is married with a two-year-old daughter. She did not say much about her husband. She presented with symptoms of depression, and she believed that no one liked her. She struggles to have her voice heard both at work and in her personal life. She is sensitive to criticism. In her family and her wider community, she feels like an outsider. Mary grew up as a Catholic in a rural part of Ireland, where she felt invisible. She described her mother as critical and judgemental of people, and she described her father as emotionally absent. Hannah wondered with Mary if she, Mary, was able to discuss any of this with her mother? Mary immediately reacted abruptly to this question and said she experienced this question as rude and intrusive. Hannah was taken aback as she had meant it in a helpful way. Hannah said she felt paralysed and was not sure how to explore this further in the next session with Mary. Elisa wondered if Mary would benefit from a DIT approach. Perhaps look at how Mary's relational patterns played out and became re-enacted with Hannah. Andrew said, 'With a CAT head on, I might ask her more explicitly about what she wanted from therapy'. These responses from Andrew and Elisa seemed somewhat intellectual to me and I wondered if the group was slipping into intellectualising and perhaps missing Mary's fragility. Like Hannah, I also felt paralysed, and I was not sure how to help the group to resonate more with Mary's fragility and Hannah's paralysis. Although we seemed to be associating freely, something defensive seemed to have emerged in the group matrix.

Peer supervision group and reflective practice

In reflecting on this supervision group in my peer supervision group, my fellow peers wondered if we had got lost in questions and answers. This peer group helpfully reminded me of the clinical hexagon and that perhaps it was important to make more use of the supervisory process rather than getting lost in the paralysis of intellectual discussion. As Smith and Gallop assert,

> the supervisor's task is to help the group move between the figure and ground of the work—what is in the forefront of their minds and what is in the background. An example would be monitoring how far their conversation focuses on the therapy and how far it may reflect their own process. Supervision group members' conversations, feelings and behaviour are potential sources of information as they reflect on their work.
>
> (Smith and Gallop, 2023: 86)

The 'clinical hexagon' speaks of the power of reflective practice, the power of free association and what Scanlon refers to as 'reflection in action' (Scanlon, 2000: 196). It offers a compass for the supervisor who can use it to think about when to intervene and where to focus, enabling both the supervisor and the supervisee to examine the therapeutic work presented in a reflective and focused manner. In reflecting on the above session, I felt better equipped for supervising the next group supervision session, which was a review session that the group had agreed to have after six months.

Vignette 3 (review)

Andrew began by saying that he was experiencing the group as a safe and important space to talk about his clinical work. He said he was beginning to realise the importance of being ordinary with his patients and not having to get it right and perfect all the time. He said, 'There's a freedom in being ordinary'. He went on to say that he had also found the group very challenging, and he worried about what the qualified therapists thought of him as he is only a psychiatrist with a limited amount of therapeutic training. Elisa said she could relate to Andrew's anxieties and said that she felt the group was helping her to feel her way through the work rather than just thinking. Hannah said she enjoyed the different approaches and that last week when Elisa mentioned DIT for her patient, she found this very helpful as it made her reflect on her own training in DIT and her therapeutic toolbox which also included coaching models, and she was pleased to be reminded of this.

I left this group feeling we had a good review and I looked forward to the next supervision after the Christmas break. However, after the Christmas break Hannah missed a session with no message. The group was left wondering about her absence and whether it was in any way related to her presentation of her patient Mary. In adhering to the group analytic concept of dynamic administration I contacted Hannah via email to check that she was ok and to say that the group had missed her. Hannah wrote back apologising for her absence and explained that she had had a family bereavement and that she would return to the group the following week. The next week Hannah did return to the group, and the following vignette describes the session:

Vignette 4

Hannah said her elderly aunt had died leaving her feeling enormously bereft. She was very close to her aunt. She had now returned to work but was struggling to focus.

    Hannah presented first—she wanted to bring back her patient Mary whom she had presented previously. She said she found the last supervision helpful, particularly what Elisa had to say about DIT. She said, 'We've now clarified what she wants from therapy—that is to say she wants to feel more confident at work and in her personal life'. She described a recent session where Mary had told her more about her husband, an older man who is prone to bouts of depression and pessimism. She added that he was currently not working and this frustrated her. Mary said that, like her mother, she tends to compartmentalise and categorise people with a moralistic lens—she compares people, she makes assumptions, binary assumptions with nothing in between. She said that she had internalised this from her parents. She cannot take or absorb compliments and she is a perfectionist. She cannot take joy from things. She believes she is unlikeable and unloveable.

Towards the end of this one-to-one session, Hannah suggested to Mary that maybe she should check out her assumptions by asking people about themselves. Mary replied, 'I feel like you are putting me in a corner when you ask this'. She then became upset and tearful. Hannah said, 'This reaction quite surprised me'.

SUPERVISOR: 'Let's check what Andrew and Elisa are thinking and feeling as they listen.'

ELISA: 'I feel warm towards her tonight.'

HANNAH: 'Yes, she did feel very authentic in this session.'

SUPERVISOR: 'I'm wondering about her tears, her upset?'

HANNAH: 'Perhaps she felt I judged her?'

ANDREW: 'I think her emotion speaks to the trust she has in you ... her tears feel positive to me.'

HANNAH: 'What do you think you feel the emotion could be? It was in response to my question ... perhaps she heard it as me being a critical parent?'

ANDREW: 'Perhaps she felt someone recognised her need? To be seen in therapy is painful. I'm feeling a sense of relief in her.'

HANNAH: 'I still think she heard it as critical.'

ELISA: 'Maybe check out with her next week—model something to her ... I think she's defending against her vulnerability.'

ANDREW: 'Mm ... I'm not sure ...'

ELISA: 'You're older than her, aren't you ... are you the critical mother in the transference? Or are you the holding mother she can't bear?'

ANDREW: 'She sounds very lonely.'

HANNAH: 'I think she is lonely and I think she is contemptuous of people including her husband ... she describes him as being like her mother—detached—but I also think she's dismissive of her husband ... and I also notice that she doesn't speak about her two-year-old daughter.'

ANDREW: 'I wonder how she experiences her daughter; in fact, I wonder if she "experiences" her daughter?'

SUPERVISOR: 'Something of an emptiness, as if there is no interconnectedness in her life.'

HANNAH: 'Yes, there is no joy in her family and so often her responses to me are subdued.'

SUPERVISOR: 'Hannah, I'm just thinking that if I was experiencing no joy in my countertransference, I would wonder about your transference to me?'

HANNAH: 'I think in the transference, I experience her as controlling—she reminds me of my friend who lives in New York—a woman who is extroverted and playful but someone who controls me, but I look forward to seeing her and I look forward to seeing Mary. They're both awkward when asked what they would like? This is Mary's second time in therapy with me.

ELISA: 'So what brought her back to therapy?'

HANNAH: 'She said she wants to be more assertive—she can't get her voice heard in groups ... she tends to feel invisible as she did when she was child growing up in Ireland.'

SUPERVISOR: 'I wonder what's happening in this group—I wonder, Hannah if you feel like you're being heard? I notice that I'm struggling to keep up with all that's been said.'

ANDREW: 'I'm now feeling dissociated. I'm also feeling this patient as empty, perhaps empty on the inside but hard or concrete on the outside.'

HANNAH: 'That's an interesting comment.'

[*Long silence.*]

ELISA: 'You're grieving Hannah—perhaps it's still really difficult for you to focus and to tune in.'

SUPERVISOR: 'And perhaps we're struggling to tune in to Hannah—I'm conscious Hannah that you've missed the last two sessions and perhaps it's hard for us to tune into you in this group?'

HANNAH: 'Well, yes, like Mary I find groups very challenging—like her, I feel inadequate ... you're all very experienced and I regard you highly but I'm afraid I'm not enough for you—perhaps I haven't described the patient enough?'

ANDREW: 'That resonates with me ... as a psychiatrist who is an unqualified psychotherapist, I feel very inadequate.'

HANNAH: 'That's what Mary speaks about in her sessions. She feels inadequate most of the time.'

I left this group with mixed feelings. On the one hand, I felt like I had allowed the group to 'free associate' and make use of their reverie. With my 'reflective practice' mind, I was keen to allow the supervisees to co-create with me and with each other while I paid attention to my own countertransference in terms of feelings, thoughts and bodily sensations. As I invited the group to reflect on what was happening in this group, Elisa associated with Hannah's difficulty in 'tuning in' and Andrew and I seemed to enter an almost manic state, resonant of Mary's state of mind. Hannah then opened up about her fear of groups, speaking to the competition and rivalry present in the group matrix. Parker reflects on the group sibling matrix, describing it as 'fundamental and intrinsic to our sense of self' (Parker, 2020: 2). The group as the medium for supervision seemed to be very active in this session.

On the other hand, I was worried that I had not fully appreciated Hannah's anxiety, both in her clinical work and in her membership of the supervision group. The next day, Hannah sent me an email saying that she had felt heard and supported the night before. Again, I was left with mixed feelings about this. As I felt Hannah was being authentic in her gratitude, I also wondered if she was in fact angry with me for describing her patient as 'empty'. In her email she alluded to feeling uncomfortable with this comment. I encouraged Hannah to bring all of this to the next session.

In discussing this group in my peer supervision group, there were also various feelings about my responses to Hannah. I felt frustrated that one of my fellow supervisees was overwhelming me with ideas and suggestions paralleling something of the strong feeling present in my supervision group and resonant of Mary's frustration in her relationship to Hannah. As I, and one of my fellow supervisees, began to acknowledge our rivalry and competition with each other, I felt freed up to notice the competition in my supervision group and my need to compete with my supervisees. This was a difficult thing for me to learn, putting me in touch with my own unconscious need to be liked and validated, replicating something of my relationships with my own siblings, which have shades of competition and rivalry. I have one brother and three sisters. My peer supervision group consisted of three women and two men. There was something about Mary's material which touched a fragile part of all group members, including me. As my peer supervision group began to look at how our own fragile selves felt misunderstood, I felt more able to understand the fragilities of my supervisees, particularly Hannah and her fear of groups, Andrew's feeling of inadequacy and Elisa's need to be perfect. Although painful, I was, with the help of both groups, able to revisit some old wounds in respect of my own family dynamic, which is always a work in progress. Parker provides a helpful description of sibling relationships never existing in isolation.

> The sibling matrix is not a fixed entity; it is an active and vibrant collection of experiences. Relationships between brothers and sisters are simply a particular perspective in a fluid inter-relational milieu.
>
> (Parker, 2020: 112)

At our next supervision group meeting, Hannah spoke about her email to me and how she felt vulnerable in presenting Mary. She admitted that she was angry with me for commenting on Mary being 'empty'. I felt a relief that there was now room for the negative transference in my supervision group. Elisa said she felt that Hannah was holding the vulnerability for the group, that is, Hannah was the person in the group who was most able to tune in to vulnerability. Andrew said he had thought more about Mary's fragility and that it made him think about his own patients who were similarly defended as Mary, that is, they appeared guarded about what they said. He said he had also thought about his own defences, and he hoped he could be more vulnerable in the group going forward. Elisa agreed and said that she was grateful to Hannah for helping her to think about her competitive nature and the impact of this on others, including her patients. Elisa also admitted that sibling rivalry is often stirred up for her in groups. She added that she realised she did not have to rely so much on my input and that I do not have all the answers.

It felt to me that the supervision group culture had turned a corner. As I too felt more in touch with my own vulnerability and fragility, I felt more at ease in my role as supervisor and subsequently more authoritative and less competitive. Foulkes asserts, 'in group analysis, and to a growing extent in psychoanalysis, we realise that the social and cultural element is deeply ingrained in the individual and is, to a large extent, unconscious' (Foulkes 1990: 163). As the group members in both supervision groups engaged in a culture of curiosity and inquiry, deeper connections evolved, not least of all between Hannah and Mary.

In the following sessions, Hannah reported that she was feeling more relaxed working with Mary. She felt more able to use her countertransference in understanding Mary's mother's transference to her. In addition, I noticed Andrew and Elisa more open to receiving feedback from me and others in the supervision group. I also noticed that I am was not so idealised, and I began to enjoy my own developing capacity to sit back and trust the group process rather than feeling a need to provide answers to the various dilemmas presented in the group. As I and my supervisees began to embody a more benign sense of authority, it emerged that Mary and other patients presented also seem able to own their own authority, feeling less persecuted in professional and personal relationships.

Conclusion

In working with the group as the medium for supervision, I felt refreshed and renewed in my group analytic attitude and thinking. The group analytic model of supervision allowed me to grow and develop both as a clinical supervisor and as a group analyst. I think the conceptual framework of 'matrix and reverie' is a powerful concept that can be applied in group supervision.

Berman and Berger comment that supervision entails creating an asymmetrical relationship between the supervisor and the supervisee. This reality, they say, tends to accrue unconscious meanings that have to do with power, hierarchies, control and dependency, and increases the supervisee's vulnerabilities.

The process of supervision, although directed towards professional growth, taps one's identity in a very personal way, and may become a source of very touchy and painful narcissistic issues. If this dynamic takes place in a supervision group, the supervisee in the group may feel 'alone, uncovered, and vulnerable, whereas all others remain comfortably dressed' (Altfeld, 1999, as cited by Berman and Berger, 2007: 239). With the help of my peer supervision group and my application of the clinical hexagon, it seemed to me that, within my supervision group, Hannah and her patient Mary no longer had to feel so anxious and overwhelmed. As the culture of competition moved to a culture of curiosity, supervisees felt more enabled to work with their differences rather than competing. In this way, deeper connections evolved in the recognition of our similarities, particularly around our shared history of not feeling good enough.

When Bion's notion of reverie and Foulkes' concept of the matrix are bound together, group supervision can enable supervisees to feel held and contained by the supervisor and by the group in a way that also enables patients to feel they are understood by their therapist. In my experience of the group presented, these same concepts also allowed the group culture to move from hierarchy and competition to one of democracy and authority.

References

Altfeld DA (1999) An experiential group model for psychotherapy supervision. *International Journal of Group Psychotherapy*, 49 (2): 237–254.

Behr H and Hearst L (2005) *Group-analytic psychotherapy: A meeting of minds.* Whurr Publishers.

Berman A and Berger M (2007) Special Section: Matrix and Reverie in Supervision Groups. *Group Analysis*, 40 (2): 236–250.

Bion WR (1962) The Psycho-Analytic Study of Thinking. *International Journal of Psychoanalysis*, 43: 306–310.

Crawford S (2005) Free Association and Supervision. In: Driver C and Martin E (eds), *Supervision and the Analytic Attitude.* Whurr Publishers.

Foulkes SH (1964) *Therapeutic Group Analysis.* George Allen and Unwin.

Foulkes SH (1990) *Selected Papers: Psychoanalysis and Group Analysis.* Routledge.

Noack A (2009) *Using the Group as a Medium of Supervision.* Supervision Review. *Journal of the British Association for Psychoanalytic and Psychodynamic Supervision.* Spring 2009, Special edition on Groups.

Parker V (2020) *A Group-Analytic Exploration of the Sibling Matrix: How Siblings Shape our Lives.* Routledge.

Plant R and Smith ME (2012) The Clinical Hexagon in Group Analytic Supervision. *The Psychotherapist*, 50: 14–15.

Scanlon C (2000) The Place of Clinical Supervision in the Training of Group-Analytic Psychotherapists: Towards a Group-Dynamic Model for Professional Education? *Group Analysis*, 33 (2): 193–207.

Searles HF (1955) The Informational Value of the Supervisor's Emotional Experiences. *Psychiatry*, 18 (2): 135–146.

Smith M (2019) Through a Glass Darkly: Using a Reflecting Team Approach in the Development of Supervisory Practice. *Group Analysis*, 52(3): 297–312. doi:10.1177/0533316419839007.

Smith M and Gallop M (2023) *Group Analytic Supervision*. Routledge.

Smith M and Plant R (2012). Group Supervision: Moving in a New Range of Experience. *The Psychotherapist*, 50: 14–15.

Winnicott DW (1971) *Playing and Reality*. Penguin Books.

Chapter 3

Narcissistic Investment as an Anti-Group Phenomenon

Fiona Pope

Setting the scene

The primary goal of therapeutic supervision is the wellbeing of the clients the therapist is working with or is planning to work with.

> Supervision is a learning process in which the psychotherapist engages with a more experienced practitioner in order to enhance his skills in the process of his ongoing professional development. This, in turn, promotes and safeguards the well-being of his clients.
>
> (Gilbert and Evans, 2000: 1)

This goal is achieved when the supervisor and the supervisee co-create a space in which the supervisee can reflect on their own wellbeing, integrate their personal development, draw on and expand their knowledge and develop their skills. All of this taking place while examining the supervisee's relationship and engagement with individual clients.

Supervisors are influenced by a number of factors, conscious and unconscious, that motivate them to enter into the work of therapeutic supervision. Conscious motivation might include a desire to support the development of therapists in training or newly qualified therapists, a hope of passing on some of their own experience and skills to their peers, a drive to raise standards within their own therapeutic setting or within the wider profession, or a means of increasing their income by accessing higher paid work.

The unconscious motivations of supervisors who decide to take on this role are probably as varied as the number of supervisors. Unconscious motivation might include providing supervision as a way of channelling the supervisor's need to care for or feel useful to others, providing supervision as a way of meeting the supervisor's own needs for relationships, avoiding burnout by reducing their exposure to direct work with clients, or maybe providing supervision as a way of creating a 'legacy' in their supervisees, i.e. by passing on their wisdom to them and thereby navigating their own fears of mortality.

DOI: 10.4324/9781032719085-4

Narcissistic investment

This chapter focuses on one specific motivation of the supervisor, that of narcissistic investment and its impact in the provision of effective group supervision in particular.

In their book, *The Supervisory Encounter*, Jacobs, David and Mayer (1995) explore the ways in which the supervisor's narcissistic self benefits from the therapeutic relationship and the role of being the supervisor. They note that narcissistic investment can arise when a supervisor feels 'fulfilled by a job well done' or fulfilled by 'the relationships with supervisees, wishing to inspire admiration or awe'. It can be evident where 'excessive investment in the supervisee's growth [is] seen as a reflection upon one's own supervisory skill', or where 'investment in the patients' progress' gives rise to the supervisor 'feeling that [the] therapeutic progress confirms the competence of the supervisee and, therefore, of the supervision' (Jacobs et al., 1995: 229).

The supervisor's narcissistic investment is satisfied by being seen by supervisees as an authority who has a bountiful supply of wisdom, knowledge and expertise. The supervisor may luxuriate in being the one who challenges the work of others, rather than having their own practice held up for scrutiny. They may inspire admiration from their supervisees, and they may even receive feelings of love and affection from them. The supervisor might experience feelings of success by proxy, from seeing the achievements of their supervisees and their clients as their own successes.

But it is not only supervisors who are potentially motivated by narcissistic investment, so too are supervisees. In *The Shadow and the Counsellor*, Steve Page writes about the motivations of counsellors:

> In the early years of being a counsellor a recognition of such factors as a desire to emulate those who have been helpful to us, the wish to help others, or a sense of calling may suffice. Gradually other, perhaps less palatable, factors start to be uncovered: the need to be needed, a perhaps slightly macabre curiosity that borders on voyeurism, an enjoyment in the sense of being important for our clients.
>
> (Page, 1999: 12)

And it is not just in the early years of practice that therapists can feel this way. Many experienced therapists are wedded to an idea of being helpful, i.e. good. Their enthusiasm about their practice is conveyed to clients in the form of empathy and optimism, and clients reinforce their approach by providing them with plenty of positive feedback, both explicit and implicit. This can have the impact of amplifying the therapists' own short comings and the deficits in their relational lives both past and present. This further heightens the therapists' narcissistic investment in the work.

When the narcissistic investment of the supervisor and the supervisee coincide, it can create an environment in therapeutic supervision where things become safe or comfortable. The needs of both parties are conveyed unconsciously to each other and there is the possibility of collusion in the relationship to such an extent that nothing is done that challenges the narcissistic investment of the other.

This situation can be further magnified when supervision takes place in a setting or context that also has a degree of narcissistic investment. This might, for example, be a charity or non-government organisation whose aims are to do 'good works' on behalf of a specific part of a local community, or it might be in a counselling service underpinned by a particular religious or faith community.

The result is an increased possibility that the supervisor and supervisee collude unconsciously to reinforce their narcissistic investment. This is not to say that the relationship would be without conflict or difficulty, but rather that disturbances or ruptures in the work are acted on or managed in such a way as to avoid challenging the narcissistic investment. As a result, the supervisory or reflective space does not contain enough intellectual and emotional rigour to enhance the therapist's practice and ultimately improve the client's experience.

In his book, *Coasting in the Countertransference*, Hirsch (2008) explores a similar theme to narcissistic investment when he looks at the 'selfish motivations both for our work with patients and in our broader professional pursuits' (Hirsch, 2008: 1). Hirsch notices that therapeutic relationships can become fixed, i.e. that therapists have a preferred style of relating to clients that fits with their own personality, which repeatedly appears in their work.

Hirsch remains curious about these factors and how they potentially stifle therapists' development as well as outcomes for clients.

> I am certain, however, that we can never be in a mutually comfortable analytic relationship for an extended period without this indicating that something disquieting and potentially destabilizing is being avoided.
>
> (Hirsch, 2008: 56)

Even in an analysis that appears to be going quite well, analysts' efforts to deconstruct familiar equilibrium is called for. 'Such an effort is inevitably in conflict with analysts' self-interest in remaining comfortable' (Hirsch, 2008: 57). Here Hirsch highlights that challenging the status quo, whilst necessary, is often defended against as it is not in the therapist's narcissistic self-interest.

Anti-group phenomena

Therapeutic supervision is delivered in both one-to-one relationships between a supervisor and supervisee and in group settings where a supervisor works with multiple supervisees in a group, typically where group members work in the same clinical setting. Group supervision has a number of advantages over individual supervision including the ability to learn directly from other group members' work with clients, being able to receive varied insights and perspectives on client work, and being part of a collective in which group members can give support to and receive support from each other.

There can also be a number of disadvantages to receiving supervision in a group and these include feeling there is less time for each individual supervisee's caseload, a confusion of ideas received from others, competition between group members, and the emergence of challenging group dynamics. Much has been documented about group dynamics, including anti-group phenomena.

Nitsun described the anti-group as:

> the destructive aspects of groups that threatens the integrity of the group and its therapeutic development. It does not describe a static 'thing' that occurs in all groups in the same way but a set of attitudes and impulses, conscious and unconscious, that manifest themselves differently in different groups.
>
> (Nitsun, 1996: 34)

Where narcissistic investment is dominant in a supervision group and where it is further reinforced by the context in which supervision is taking place, there is the danger that the group's efforts to satisfy this narcissistic investment potentially inhibits growth and learning. And, as Nitsun wrote, the anti-group process needs 'recognition and handling in order that the constructive development of the group can proceed without serious obstruction' (Nitsun, 1996: 34).

The following examples highlight a few ways in which narcissistic investment might arise as an anti-group phenomenon in group supervision.

- The supervisor might prioritise their role as a group facilitator, i.e. focusing on being an effective manager of boundaries—allocating time and managing confidentiality—at the expense of greater creativity and exploration in the group.
- The supervisor might have a blind spot and be unable or unwilling to see anything that falls outside of a cohesive group experience, they may fail to respond to or fail to explore acts of aggression or feelings of competition within the group.
- The supervisor might take pride in the experience of facilitating a cohesive and non-conflictual group. In this way, they convey to the group members that more challenging aspects of group interactions are not welcome in the group. Group members pick up on these cues and fall in line. This may be particularly true if group members are in training and are reliant on feedback from their supervisor to obtain their qualifications. They might supress competitive feelings that arrive naturally within

a group setting or that arrive between themselves and individuals who are talented or experienced members of the group.

- A supervisor might fail to bring intellectual rigour to the group in the form of new literature, theory and research for fear of being exposed as not being up to date in these areas.
- Supervisees might also contribute to the anti-group phenomena by prioritising narcissistic investment over the effective functioning of the group. This might take place in a number of ways. For example:

a   Supervisees in the group might be more willing to offer empathy to their peers—be it for their personal life circumstances or their difficulties working with complex clients—at the expense of offering an appropriate level of feedback or challenge to less than skilful practice.

b   Supervisees might not share or might actively suppress their own feelings about other group members or regarding the presentation of a peer's client for fear that it will generate tensions in the group.

c   Supervisees might focus solely on client work and avoid dynamics that are arising in the supervision group. Supervisees may work hard to ensure that supervision is a place where clinical work is discussed and the intimacy of I-thou relating with other group members is minimised.

Nitsun went on to say that,

> I also believe that the successful handling of the anti-group represents a turning point in the development of the group. By helping the group to contain its particular anti- group, not only are the chances of destructive acting out reduced, but the group is strengthened, its survival reinforced and its creative power liberated.
>
> (Nitsun, 1996: 44)

Similarly, Hisch noted the potential to be beneficial depends largely on whether 'efforts are made to stretch oneself to areas of discomfort, thereby serving to potentially expand the analytic relationship' (Hirsch, 2008: 55). It is therefore critical to address narcissistic investment in order to manage the anti-group phenomena impacting the group's ability to perform in a mature and effective manner and complete its task.

Addressing issues of shame

One of the antidotes to narcissistic investment and its impact on group supervision comes from recognising and addressing issues of shame, both in the supervisor and the supervisees.

Christiane Sanderson has written about the importance of being able to recognise and work with shame for the benefit of clients. She describes that shame is a universal emotion that is an inevitable part of the human condition. 'Shame is a primary emotion that facilitates bonds, allowing us to connect to others and experience a sense of belonging. This is necessary for survival, prosocial behaviour, empathy and compassion' (Sanderson, 2015: 1).

She goes on to note: 'The healthy expression of shame is a powerful adaptive strategy that ensures survival and promotes affiliation. However, when shame is too harshly imposed, it can become toxic and imprison the individual in abyss of self-hate and self-blame' (Sanderson, 2015: 1).

Shame arrives whenever we are in a relationship and, in particular, when there is a component of dependency and vulnerability in the relationship—and this is equally true in therapeutic supervision and supervision groups. Sources of shame for the supervisor, in group supervision might include the following.

- Being a group supervisor is a relational activity. The supervisor's ability to make, develop and sustain relationships will arrive with the supervisory setting and the supervisor will be aware of their own shortcomings in this regard.
- Furthermore, a group supervisor has an important role as a group facilitator whether the supervision group is newly formed or well established—and again the supervisor will have an awareness of the group's competence and development needs in this area. Group supervisors might also have feelings of shame if they feel they are not able to relate to all members of the group equally.
- The feelings of shame that a supervisor might have in regard to making and managing relationships and facilitating groups will be amplified by the group, who operate as a witness to these processes in the supervisor.
- Supervisors often have a wealth of experience gained from working in a range of settings. However, they will typically be practising with less experienced supervisees who have more recently undergone therapeutic training and so may have access to more up-to-date knowledge, theoretical developments and research-based data. Supervisors can experience feelings of shame from being out of touch and their inadequacy in these areas being exposed by their supervisees.

For the supervisee, sources of shame in group supervision might include the following.

- Supervisees are dependent on their supervisor, and this brings with it an inevitable imbalance of power that generates feelings of shame.
- In supervision, a supervisee will inevitably expose their shortcomings and difficulties in their clinical work. Supervisees use supervision to reflect on their mistakes, blocks or impasses in the work and this is highly exposing.
- Supervisees can have a strong drive to be a 'perfect' practitioner. This can be accentuated if they are in training and needing to prove their abilities

to supervisors and training organisations. The flawed self might be seen as unacceptable.

- Supervisees' shame can often be invoked if their placement setting or training organisation puts unrealistic expectations on them. For example, to work with complex clients who need to work with a more experienced or more specialised practitioner. Similarly, supervisors can compound a supervisee's feelings of shame by having unrealistic expectations of their abilities and not questioning if the work is beyond their competence.
- Supervisees can feel shame in group supervision in response to a comparison and/or hierarchy that emerges in the group, based on their perception of competence, experience, expertise or likeability.
- Supervisees can also feel shame about needing to belong to the group and be accepted and included or with regard to feelings of rivalry for the attention and affection of the group supervisor.
- And, finally, it is important to note that client material and client experiences related to shame can be experienced by supervisees in their countertransference responses and these can also arrive in supervision.

Narcissistic investment can be addressed and its impact mitigated within group supervision by creating a culture of shame awareness within the group. This culture of shame awareness can be developed in a number of ways.

A supervisor who has invested time to educate themselves about the ways in which shame is generated, how shame is expressed, defences against shame and skills for working with shame will be better able to engage with their own feelings of shame and to recognise its presence in supervisees and in the group.

It is important that a supervisor is mindful of the inherent nature of shame within supervision. This includes shame generated by the power imbalance in the relationship between supervisor and supervisee as well as the shame generated by exposing mistakes or difficulties and asking for help. A supervisor can help unearth and explore feelings of shame in regard to supervision and enable it to be articulated clearly and discussed within the group, thereby preventing the feelings from going underground.

A supervisor can model the ability to manage feelings of shame by making explicit reference to their own feelings of shame and by talking openly about the limits of their experience and knowledge. Modelling ways of dealing with feelings of shame will also usefully include the supervisor's description of mistakes in their own clinical practice and ways of understanding and working with these.

A supervisor might also mitigate the impact of shame by encouraging supervisees in the group to bring their own feelings of shame into the open. This might be in regard to client work but also, where relevant, might include aspects of their own personal selves, childhood experiences, relationship difficulties and, for counsellors in training, struggles with completing coursework for training institutions. Encouragement might also take the form of providing positive feedback to group members willing to share their experiences, which in turn might enable or encourage other group members to do the same.

The supervisor can also mitigate the impact of shame by working with group dynamics and group processes, particularly those that appear to be influenced by shame, and doing so in a way that is driven from a place of being curious and exploratory rather than critical and judgemental.

It will also be important for the supervisor to be aware of the possibility that a client's shame is arriving unconsciously in the group through parallel process and might need to be disentangled from that of the supervisee.

A supervision group might also benefit from the encouragement of curiosity and play. In some circumstances this might include the use of creative approaches, techniques or materials as a means of moving away from exposure and shame and towards open exploration.

Self-esteem

As the supervisor and the supervision group recognise and address issues of shame, the impact of narcissistic investment lessens and self-esteem emerges as an alternative lens. Self-esteem refers to a person's realistic assessment of their abilities and limitations. It refers to a person's beliefs about their own worth and value. Self-esteem is important because it influences a person's choices and decisions.

Jacobs, David and Meyer describe the many ways in which a supervisor can support a supervisee's self-esteem.

> [By] empathic interest in the student's experience of therapy, validation of his competence and talent, realistic praise and admiration for his efforts and accomplishments, and encouragement of his pursuit of mastery of his skills, especially during periods of confusion, doubt, and discouragement.
> (Jacobs et al., 1995: 233)

In this way, the supervisor and other group members help the therapist see themselves more clearly. This improves self-esteem by increasing the therapist's accuracy of their perception of themselves and identifying distortions that they might have.

This realistic appraisal by the supervisee is important. It needs to include some awareness of their limitations and address 'blind spots' in their practice. Here the role of the supervisor and the supervision group is important as it helps the therapist to understand their narcissistic investment.

The critical turning point in the development of self-esteem comes from addressing narcissistic investment and its influence as an anti-group phenomenon. This comes from redirecting narcissistic investment away from getting things 'right' and towards understanding when and why things are going 'wrong'.

Jacobs, David and Meyer describe a redirection of narcissistic investment as 'Rather than feeling that one's personal-worth hinges on winning a battle, one derives satisfaction and self-esteem from the ability to understand why the battle is happening [in the first place]' (Jacobs et al., 1995: 239).

This involves the supervisor giving weight and attention to feelings of 'dis-ease' when they arrive in the group, allowing their confusion and uncertainty to arrive and trusting the group's ability to manage and hold these difficulties. In this way, the supervisor enhances the working of the group, builds the self-esteem of the participants and enables practitioners to better support their clients.

Vignette

John is a 46-year-old man who has a role as a counselling supervisor at a local charity. The charity provides low-cost, open-ended counselling to adults who are survivors of domestic violence in childhood.

John joined the service in a voluntary capacity while he was undertaking his training in group supervision. He has a private practice of clients and individual supervisees. John decided to continue to volunteer for the service as a group supervisor after he completed his training because he believes in supporting his local community and making counselling more accessible to those on low incomes.

John has experience of growing up in a household where verbal aggression from his father to his mother was the norm.

John supervises a group of three volunteer counsellors, all of whom have completed person-centred counselling training. Sophie has recently joined the group; she is studying at a Gestalt training organisation. This is Sophie's first placement, and she has talked in the group about her anxiety about the work and being keen to get things right for her clients.

Sophie attended the group on three occasions. At the fourth meeting, Archie, who has been volunteering for the organisation for five years presents a client called Muriel. Archie noted how the sessions with Muriel have improved as Muriel has moved from being very closed, withdrawn and hard to engage to more trusting and more willing to speak about her life and her childhood experiences of abuse.

Sophie responded to Archie's presentation of Muriel with some passion when she noted that Archie did not seem to be concerned about what Muriel described as her 'management' of her ten-year-old daughter. Muriel gives her daughter the 'silent treatment' and 'freezes her out' by not speaking to her for a period of 24 hours when she has done something that Muriel did not approve of.

Sophie said it felt that the therapy could not be going 'well' if a client felt better but continued to operate in an unkind, uncaring and even abusive way in their relationships. Sophie seemed agitated as she spoke and found it hard to make eye contact with Archie, while speaking with a degree of energy that Archie said he experienced as aggressive.

John took this experience to his own supervision group, wondering why Sophie might be finding it hard to fit into the group and how he might help her with this.

With the help of his supervision group, John was able to see that his main focus was on how to maintain the established and comfortable way of the group experience.

The supervisor wondered if Sophie had a point, if there wasn't a tendency in the group to present progress and to skirt over more concerning aspects in the work? The supervisor noted that when Sophie had entered the group, she was not willing to collude and overlook the potential abusive behaviour of the client.

John found himself justifying his work to his supervisor and defending himself by noting the number of years in which he had successfully run the group.

The supervisor was able to gently note that John seemed defensive and wondered if something might be being touched personally for him? John reflected and wondered if he experienced Sophie as verbally aggressive, which reminded him of his own abusive father. John expressed surprise that this material could still be activated in him. John's supervisor was able to empathise with the 'young part of John' and wondered about any feelings of shame that he might carry about his father.

John recognised feelings of hurt and disappointment related to his father. He went on to describe feelings of shame that his mother had tolerated his father's abuse and thereby left John at his mercy, in essence devaluing John. As John described this experience in supervision, he was able to see that Sophie was also a challenge to him as she had embodied a position that his mother had not been able to take with his father, and called out the behaviour.

John was able to return to the supervision group more in touch with his own experiences and feelings of shame. He started the next session by sharing his feeling of regret that he had not been better able to work with what had happened in the previous meeting with the group members and that he felt sad about that. He went on to explore with Sophie and Archie what had been touched for them personally and professionally in their exchange.

Sophie was able to describe her feelings of anger about the situation. This opened up the opportunity for the group to wonder where the client's anger might be, how it gets expressed and if there were ways Muriel might want to do that differently without being punishing to her daughter. Archie was able to notice the feelings of exposure he felt when Sophie highlighted something that he felt he had 'missed' in the client work. He described feeling vulnerable and fearful of what this meant for his position in the group and in John's eyes, whose opinion he valued highly.

Archie returned to the supervision group two weeks later and presented his work with Muriel again. He noted that he had wondered with Muriel how she felt after the difficult exchanges with her daughter. Muriel described that while initially she felt her silences were justified, as time wore on, she felt more embarrassed about what she was doing and out of control of the situation and relationship with her daughter. Archie and Muriel had begun to explore what alternatives might be open to her at points of conflict with her daughter.

In this work, John, Sophie and Archie were all able to move away from positions that were about 'getting it right', doing therapy 'properly' and maintaining the status quo in the group. They avoided scapegoating each other. As John was able to engage with his own feelings of shame and defensiveness and explore the impact of his own shortcomings, he enabled the group to work through a rupture, learn more about each other and recalibrate what the client might need or benefit from exploring.

Conclusion

One of the antidotes to narcissistic investment that operates as an anti-group phenomenon in group supervision is the creation of a culture of shame awareness. This helps redirect narcissistic investment away from getting things right and towards understanding when and how things go wrong. Through engagement in this way the individual supervisee is able to explore blind spots and develop their insight, knowledge and skill. Furthermore, the group becomes a place where rupture and difficulty can be explored and resolved. This is turn builds self-esteem.

References

Gilbert M and Evans K (2000) *Psychotherapy Supervision*. Open University Press.

Hirsch I (2008) *Coasting in the Countertransference: Conflicts of Self Interest Between Analyst and Patient* (1st ed.). Routledge.

Jacobs D, David P and Meyer D (1995) *The Supervisory Encounter: A Guide for Teachers of Psychodynamic Psychotherapy and Psychoanalysis*. Yale University Press.

Nitsun M (1996) The Concept of the Anti-Group. *The Anti-Group: Destructive Forces in the Group and Their Creative Potential*. Routledge, pp. 42–74.

Page S (1999) *The Shadow and the Counsellor*. Routledge.

Sanderson C (2015) *Counselling Skills for Working with Shame*. Jessica Kingsley Publishers.

Chapter 4

Dreams and Supervision[1]

Amelie Noack

> We are such stuff as dreams are made on …
>> (Shakespeare, *The Tempest*, 1611: Act 4, scene 1, 156–158)

Putting dreams and supervision together under one heading creates a rather complex picture. There are the patients' dreams and how one works with them in supervision; there is working with dreams about supervision or the supervisor see (Vaslamatzis, 1993); and we also have Ogden's idea that good supervision is about establishing a dreamlike state of reverie in supervision in order for supervisor and supervisee to 'dream up' the patient (Ogden, 2005).

Dreaming about patients

A further facet of this complexity would be a therapist's dreams about their patients and how to address these in supervision. Bringing my dreams about one of my patients to supervision as a trainee turned into a rather difficult experience at the time, because my supervisor said that this showed that I had not kept safe boundaries. I ended up feeling extremely guilty. In retrospect my guilt appears rather puzzling, especially because nowadays I do expect my patients to 'intrude' into my psychic space in order for me to comprehend and eventually understand their psychic experience more fully. Projective identifications into the analyst's mind are what defines and fundamentally informs the therapeutic process. We usually understand and actively use the information gleaned that way as countertransference information and apply these insights in the work with the patient. I am sure each reader has examples of this from their own experience.

However, during the early stage of one of my periods of training, I faithfully reported the dreams I had of a patient in supervision, hoping to gain further insight into their psychic functioning. Instead, my supervisor told me that I had to learn to protect myself better from my patient's intrusive manoeuvres. My supervisor was adamant that I was too sensitive, and I ended up feeling that I had failed the patient by allowing them to 'intrude' into my own psychic space. My dilemma at the time originated without doubt in the

DOI: 10.4324/9781032719085-5

difficulties I experienced in the relationship with my supervisor. I had been expecting support and clarification and had hoped for help to develop my understanding as a professional further. I had known that this would also include challenges but, in the event, it seemed that I could not get anything right. I experienced the supervisor's attitude as punitive and their responses to my work seemed full of negative feedback and criticism. I became afraid of each supervision session and felt increasingly insecure and a failure.

Colman suggests that psychotherapists always feel vulnerable in their work, because 'feelings of anxiety, guilt and inadequacy can be felt as personal failings, but they are inevitable aspects of psychoanalytic work' (Colman, 2006: 100). He continues to say that this dilemma is worsened through the contamination of the feelings of anxiety, guilt and inadequacy by judgemental intolerance and condemnation, deriving from a persecutory superego attitude. Analytic failings are then often projected onto other colleagues, while analytic superiority is identified with and vice versa, to such a degree that a persecutory superego may well define the speck in a colleague's eye as their inability to see. These processes can be damaging especially during training. The persecutory superego function can be projected onto the training institution and onto the trainers, as well as supervisors—but again, trainers and supervisors themselves might well identify with a cruel superego and behave in a persecutory way. Colman points out that the supervisor plays a decisive role in that respect, because his or her attitude will determine whether a trainee can use the supervisor as a mediator to become less fearful of persecution (Colman, 2007). To realise an attitude of open-mindedness, curiosity, free play and creativity, which are essential for successful therapeutic work, is a real accomplishment. Here the supervisor can make the difference and help to replace the harsh superego constraints of a persecutory superego with ego judgement, so that 'boundaries can become lodged not in rules but in the analyst's own thinking mind' (Colman, 2006: 99).

As it happened, though, the work with this particular training supervisor became increasingly unbearable. My persecutory anxieties grew, and each supervision session seemed a nightmare, so that I finally requested to change supervisors. This decision felt somewhat dangerous and had the consequence that my qualification was delayed. Now, many years later, I am glad I was able to make this decision. There was a price to pay, but the thinking behind my assessment has become part of my own development as a clinician. In the wake of these experiences, I discovered that supervision can be understood and experienced as an interactional event and that, on this basis, the supervisee themself 'must … quietly monitor the status and qualities of his or her supervisor's work' (Langs, 1994: 208). This has informed my personal style as a supervisor. Moreover, the experience also provided the impulse for my endeavour to understand the supervisory process more fully.

Supervision as dreaming

Some time ago, I had the opportunity to observe some supervisory work through a one-way mirror. This work was done as part of the supervision course at the Institute of Group Analysis in London. As a member of a small group observing a second small group during a supervisory session, we were outside the room and could see the supervision group through the one-way mirror while the sound was transferred to us outside the room through a transmitter. The people in the supervision group were speaking, asking questions and responding to each other. We could hear and understand what went on. After some time, however, the sound of the voices became quieter and quieter, so much so, that it was eventually difficult for all of us outside the supervision room to hear what was said. We could now only hear mumbling voices, while the supervision went on. While we could still see people talking, for us 'outsiders' there seemed to be an increasing silence. The events on the other side of the one-way mirror were to us 'shrouded' in a dreamlike stillness. After this, we observed another supervision group, also through the one-way mirror, and this time we could hear the group well throughout the allotted time. Afterwards, in the following discussion amongst all the groups, it became apparent that the first supervision group had not been aware of the decrease in their sound level at all. Interestingly enough, it turned out that the work being discussed so quietly related to a session with a group, where 'being seen but not heard' had been a topic for a patient. The patient still found it difficult to speak up, to make themselves heard and to feel heard.

I would like to make a connection between this experience and the way proposed by Ogden (2005) for working in supervision. In his view, it is the task of the supervisor to create a frame—or a facilitating environment, as I might call it in reference to Winnicott (1960)—in order to help the supervisee generate and sustain a receptive state of reverie. In this state of reverie, the patient can be 'dreamed' by the analyst. Based on the analyst's unconscious, preconscious and conscious experiences of the patient, when in supervision, both supervisor and supervisee participate in this process, which brings to life the therapeutic work in the supervisory relationship itself, in that supervisor and supervisee together will 'dream up' the patient. Working in supervision in this way, Ogden says, can become like dreaming. It depends on the supervisor's capacity to create a secure frame, fostering a sense of honesty and intimacy, and allowing the use of reverie and free association.

This, I believe, throws light on what had happened on the supervision course. It seemed to me that the first supervision group moved increasingly into a dreamlike state, 'dreaming up' the patient. In contrast, our observing group outside the supervision room and outside the supervisory space, stayed awake, observed and could point out afterwards what had been happening.

Dreaming—a universal language

In his book *The Forgotten Language*, Erich Fromm tells us that dreams, myths and fairy tales are all made of the same stuff (Fromm, 1991). And we human beings are too made of this stuff, as one of the great storytellers of humanity, Shakespeare, tells us.

All over the world, people dream dreams, in which the decisive elements and events in human life take form—the pleasures, the catastrophes and the miracles and wonders of living. After dying in a dream, I can 'wake up', like Sleeping Beauty, discovering that I am still alive. After the ugly sisters cut off their toes to fit into Cinderella's slipper, they are still as ugly and envious, when I read the story the next time. In every myth or epos (a poem containing local traditions), the hero—whether it is Gilgamesh or Superman—combats evil and attempts to win the treasure. The various stories have their different cultural overlay, since lives lived in Africa or Iceland are different. The stories may appear new, like Harry Potter's trials and tribulations, or they may be 3,000 years old. The images, fantasies, ideas and symbols give evidence of a universal language spoken by our human imagination.

Stories, fairy tales and myths—all arise from a universal level of psychic functioning pertaining to all of humanity, a layer of psyche which is common to us all. According to Jung, this layer of the unconscious, where symbols, images and energies reside, is the collective unconscious (Jung, 1977). He describes dreams as the 'little hidden door in the innermost and most secret recesses of the soul opening into that cosmic night which was psyche long before there was any ego-consciousness, and which will remain psyche no matter how far our ego-consciousness may extend ... It is from these all-uniting depths that the dream arises be it ever so childish, grotesque, and immoral' (Jung, 1953: 46).

The group analyst Foulkes also refers to this deep layer of the unconscious and called it the foundation matrix (Foulkes, 1990). The matrix as such is a group analytic concept describing the communicative and interactive conscious and unconscious processes between the members of a given group. The foundation matrix itself describes the deepest layer of this matrix and is based on the 'socialness' of humans. This deep layer is the common shared ground of any group and includes the phylogenetic heritage of being human, including a store of shared communication and meaning preceding every actual group. This fundamental mental matrix also contains affect expressions, since basic affects are innate and shared by all humanity and can be understood and communicated very early in life by all humans (Scholz, 2003). This has now been substantiated through recent neurophysiological research, which found, amongst other aspects, so-called mirror neurons in the brain, which allow for mutual action understanding between human beings.

Besides images, the foundation matrix contains also aspects of language, social class and education, and these aspects vary from culture to culture.

Every culture contains in its matrix deprecations of other cultures, as well as the international history and their power relations (Scholz, 2004). I believe this point is especially important to acknowledge in the multicultural societies we now live in. Multicultural groups with their variety of backgrounds, including class, sexual orientation, ethnicity or culture, have a high potential for insecurity since they have a smaller shared common ground. The underlying differences and cultural variations between people with other sexual or gender orientations or from other countries (like visitors, refugees or asylum-seekers) generate a greater base of general anxiety and aggression. We need to learn to recognise these differences and address and think about them. This is a task for all educational institutions, including the training institutes for therapists. The deep and often unconscious mutual cultural deprecations, which may be encountered on the path to mutual understanding and acceptance, throw light on the difficulties that are part and parcel of therapeutic and supervisory work. If understood and worked with appropriately, they can help to develop a value system that embraces diversity and invites otherness. While our dreams may all come from the same source, in a multicultural setting we may well regard each other as strangers or even enemies, standing on opposite sides of the river, seemingly threatening to each other.

The attempt to enter a state of reverie, where we may touch on each other's dreams, as described by Ogden as a model for supervision, may be one way to build a bridge across the river, not just between analyst and patient, supervisor and supervisee, but also between different sexual and gender orientations, between classes, cultures and nationalities. We all are dreamers.

In 'social dreaming', dreams are used for the purpose of building bridges (Lawrence, 2005): a group of strangers can share their dreams, without interpreting but by associating with the dreams. This allows a dreamlike and somewhat egoless state to develop, which creates a space for new links to be made and new meaning to emerge. Social dreaming offers a chance to make connections in our attempt to relate to our shared common ground. It allows us to build bridges projecting into space, to something that could not be thought about before, on the way to a greater mutual understanding of each other as human beings.

Dreaming supervision

True to the idea of dreaming, I have allowed myself to meander a bit in this paper. My conclusion is that there is no one recipe for working with dreams in supervision. It takes time and trust to work with dreams, as it takes trust and time to develop a good supervisory relationship, not just with our supervisees, but also with our own self-reflective capacities.

One of my therapy groups loves bringing dreams. At some point, I realised that there had been no dreams recently—and that I had not properly addressed this. I wondered if my work with the group's dreams had been lacking and if I had even felt a bit helpless about how to work with them. While I pondered this, two people told one dream each in the next session. Both dreams seemed really important, and I decided that I would write them down later, after the session. But to my utter dismay I could only remember one of the dreams. It was obviously significant that I could not remember the second dream, I was missing something essential. The evening before the next session I was thinking about all this again, but could still not remember any more detail, nor did I feel any further understanding.

The following day, early in the session, another group member asked for the second dream to be retold, because, as they said, they had felt unable to remember it. Others nodded and both dreams were retold then. I listened carefully. The first dreamer said their dream was about 'an ending, which could mean either success or failure, which one was not clear'. The second dreamer reported that they had dreamt about 'a world-destroying catastrophe, a disaster' and that they had woken in terror and had not been able to go back to sleep for a considerable time afterwards. After a short silence the group member who had asked to hear the dreams again said to the second dreamer: 'No wonder I could not remember your dream.' We all nodded.

After a while the group took up the theme of catastrophe of the second dream. Each group member spoke about experiences in their lives where they had suffered through something akin to disaster. The whole group was engaged, and every group member contributed with one or more examples from their own experience. These were difficult and painful stories, and the group listened intently. Going through something like a catastrophe obviously had different meanings for every member of the group. Then it happened that one group member mentioned that all these stories of disaster were in the past, that they all had an ending of some kind. This prompted the group to move in their discussion increasingly between both dreams, elucidating an aspect from their experience of disaster with aspects from the second dream about ending. It seemed that the encounter with disaster could only begin to become tolerable and be thought about when it was connected with the other, more palatable, dream. The experience of an ending, with the open question of whether that meant success or failure, seemed to offer a counterpart to living through catastrophe in the other dream. Imagining an ending made it possible to start digesting disaster.

The group members resonated with each other's stories and contributed to different aspects of both dreams. During this to-ing and fro-ing a tapestry of meaning developed in the group and allowed a growing understanding of the aspects of each dream in regard to each group member's history and life. It seemed a very rich and thoughtful session. This session also demonstrates the process though which unthinkable elements of experience are transformed, so that experience that can begin to be processed and eventually develop into thoughts that can begin to be thought about. This clearly resonates with Bion's ideas (Bion, 1984). While a member of my group could dream of a world-destroying catastrophe and tell the dream in the group, other people in the group, including myself, could not remember the dream. We had not been able to allow the dream access into our psychic space, because it was too terrifying. It *had* to be forgotten, and so could not be remembered. A dream of the end of the world is certainly the stuff of nightmares, but it may also border on what Ogden calls night terrors. Ogden declares that night terrors are dreams that cannot yet be dreamed, let alone thought about (Ogden, 2005).

I believe that this intense piece of work only became possible for the group, because I had noticed and acknowledged the lack of focus on dreams. I felt concerned about the group and helpless—and in a somewhat self-supervisory capacity I admitted that something was amiss. I allowed myself to become preoccupied with the group and dreaming—in parallel with Winnicott's notion of maternal preoccupation—and my lack of understanding. This allowed a change to occur in the therapeutic space and made it possible for something new to emerge.

It is our bodies that dream, not our conscious egos. Dreaming is an activity of our whole being and can be understood as the attempt to digest and process intense, difficult and even traumatic emotional experience. Fairy tales and their stories about tricky personal situations give examples of how to deal with these difficulties on an individual level. The heroes in our myths provide solutions for society in general or for a particular culture, by proposing ideas and offering illustrations for how to think about collective difficulties or trauma, like, for instance, losing a war or a people's chosen trauma. This deep level of human functioning, where biology, sociology and psychology all meet, is under constant construction through communication, action and interaction by humanity as a whole, in conscious and unconscious ways. In that depth of psyche, where our bodies and minds connect, and boundaries between self and other blur or even go altogether at times, new developments are being forged and sometimes emerge in our dreams.

Note

1 This paper is a revised version of an article first published in Supervision Review— *The Journal of the British Association for Psychoanalytic and Psychodynamic Supervision*, Spring 2010: 12–18.

References

Bion WR (1984) *Second Thoughts*. Karnac Books.
Colman W (2006) The Analytic Superego. *Journal of the British Association of Psychotherapists*, 42: 99–114.
Colman W (2007) The Supervisor and the Super-Ego. *Newsletter of the British Association for Psychoanalytic and Psychodynamic Supervision*. www.interscience.com. doi:10.1002/bap.107.

Foulkes SH (1990) *Selected Papers of SH Foulkes: Psychoanalysis and Group Analysis.* Karnac Books.

Fromm E (1991) *The Forgotten Language: An Introduction to the Understanding of Dreams, Fairy Tales and Myths.* Evergreen.

Jung CG (1953) *Psychological Reflections.* Panther.

Jung CG (1977) *Symbols of Transformation (Collected Works of C.G. Jung).* Princeton University Press.

Langs R (1994) *Doing Supervision and Being Supervised.* Karnac Books.

Lawrence WG (2005) *Introduction to Social Dreaming, Transforming Thinking.* Karnac Books.

Ogden TH (2005) On Psychoanalytic Supervision. *International Journal of Psychoanalysis,* 86(5): 1265–1280.

Scholz R (2003) The Foundation Matrix—A Useful Fiction. *Group Analysis,* 36: 548–554.

Scholz R (2004) Self-Esteem and the Process of its Reassessment in Multicultural Groups: Renegotiating the Symbolic Social Order. *Group Analysis,* 37 (4): 525–535.

Vaslamatzis G (1993) Some Transference-Countertransference Issues of the Supervisory Situation: A Dream About the Supervisor. In Alexandris A and Vaslamatzis G (eds), *Countertransference: Theory, Technique, Teaching.* Routledge.

Winnicott DW (1960) The Theory of the Parent-Infant Relationship. *International Journal of Pyschoanalysis,* 41: 585–595.

Part 2

Working with Difference in Group Supervision

Chapter 5

Cross-Cultural Issues in Supervision

Elisabeth Rohr

In the last decades, supervision has spread and has gained recognition way beyond clinical and psychotherapeutical fields of work. This has definitely been true for Germany and other European countries, even though there are some national differences. In Germany this development becomes evident when looking at the membership of the professional organisation Deutsche Gesellschaft für Supervision (DGSv; German Society for Supervision), which counts today more than 4,000 members (DGSv, 2008). However, it also shows in the growing number of master studies in supervision in many universities and academic institutions.

Supervision has a long tradition in Germany, especially supervision in educational, social and administrative organisations. Of course, supervision within psychotherapeutic training has always existed as an obligatory part of any psychotherapeutic training. Nevertheless, it is important to point out that supervision, as we know it today and as we practise it in Germany, has two major historical roots: psychoanalysis and social work (especially case management). Awareness of these two historical roots has had an essential and major influence on the development of supervision in Germany, since the theoretical background of supervision was not only shaped by the practice and the experience of psychoanalysis and its clinical application but also by the practice and experience of social work. Therefore, it can be assumed there are some cultural differences in the way supervision is exercised in different European countries. For example, in Germany social and educational theories have been integrated into the training of supervisors and in the shaping of theoretical and methodological concepts of supervision, namely the concepts of Bourdieu (Bourdieu, 1986 [1984]).

In the following, I focus mainly on supervision that takes place outside the clinical realm of work, mainly in educational, social and administrative organisations and then I focus on cross-cultural supervision.

Definition and aims of supervision

The German Society for Supervision defines supervision as a specific form of counselling for persons whose primary task is to work with people and who

DOI: 10.4324/9781032719085-7

therefore constantly have to reflect their own professional position in the tension between proximity and distance in relation to their clients (DGSv, n.d.).

Supervision is considered a scientifically based, practice-oriented and ethically bound concept for personal and organisational consultations within labour frameworks. It is an effective form of counselling in situations of high complexity, differentiation and dynamic change (DGSv, n.d.).

The counselling process is particularly concerned with the reflection of experiences and processes within a specific institutional context, the impact of structures, processes and organisational patterns in the behaviour of people involved, the analysis and clarification of complex interrelationships, conflict dynamics and the resolution of conflicts, and professional education and qualification processes (DGSv, n.d.).

Supervision aims at an increase of personal, social and professional capacities and at a deeper understanding of experiences and actions in diverse professional relationships and interactions, particularly in cases of problem solving in critical and complex situations (DGSv, n.d.).

Supervision is therefore always subject-, process- and context-orientated and can be described methodologically as a form of dialogue, containing multiple perspectives and offering a variety of possible results.

The basic attitude of a supervisor is characterised by appreciation and impartiality; it is resource-orientated, with personal commitment and empathy and, therefore, capable of enduring contradictions, tensions and ambiguities as well as developing new perspectives.

Finally, supervision as a profession is committed to social responsibility for education, health, fundamental rights, democracy, justice, peace and sustainable development (DGSv, n.d.).

Intercultural supervision

How do all these definitions and explanations of supervision apply to cross-cultural or culturally sensitive supervision? We begin by emphasising the importance of some culturally specific ways of dealing with time, social relationships and life in general.

Orientations within cultures

Monochronistic cultures

Tight planning of activities, agenda always has priority, interruptions cause irritations, and time is linear and precious and should not be wasted.

People living in monochronistic cultures usually do not have any major difficulties in arriving on time for supervision. Dates are fixed in their agendas and they do not have to be reminded about future dates of meetings. However, they might feel under pressure if the process does not develop rapidly, and they can feel impatient, as though they are wasting time.

Polychronic cultures

Relationships always have priority, time is flexible and agendas can always be changed; time is circular, repetitive, there will always be another chance, there is no need to hurry.

People, living in polychronistic cultures might have difficulty in understanding that it is important to be on time for the session, because there are always so many other priorities to attend to—there will always be a next time, why to submit to such rigidity (Tschetschonig, 2012)?

Dealing with social relationships

High-context cultures

Contacts are everything and social networks are essential. There are strong dependencies on families and social networks.

Low-context cultures

Documents count and facts are what matters—for example, academic degrees, educational performance, certificates (Hall, 1976). However, informal social networks or families are not there to share emotions, they are there to protect the individual and to secure the individual's belonging. To secure belonging in high-context cultures speaking about emotions should be avoided (and might cause shame). Therefore, supervision is about overcoming anxiety and shame. In low-context cultures, social status might be significant and lead to a competitive atmosphere, overshadowing an in-depth discussion of difficulties and conflicts.

Specific trans-cultural skills

Having all this in mind, in addition to the regular supervisory skills, there are a number of skills and abilities that are necessary in order to be able to work and think in a culturally heterogeneous context.

On the one hand, a fundamental cultural sensitivity is required. This goes hand in hand with a genuine interest in hybrid lifestyles, in what is alien to us in ourselves and in others. It is important here to adopt an open, but authentic attitude, to be curious about all the unknowns that surround us and that we encounter in the world, without making hasty judgements and without rash ethnocentric categorisations. This also means tolerating the unknown, the unfamiliar, without immediately pigeonholing it, simply enduring the uncertainty that it triggers.

On the other hand, we need to recognise and reflect on differences in power and hierarchy. As White Europeans, we undoubtedly have many privileges and live in a situation of social and economic luxury compared to other people in other parts of the world. This is very clearly perceived by everybody in any given transcultural context. In addition, as Germans we are confronted in almost all parts of the world, and of course also in migration-related contexts in Germany, by the Nazi past—often silently of course, but these historical and cultural transferences are immediately noticeable when we identify ourselves as Germans. It is important neither to ignore nor to deny these cultural transferences, but to take note of them and address them when the opportunity arises. This gives us authenticity and sincerity and helps us in our supervisory work, since we make it clear that it is important to talk about 'secrets' in order to address difficult issues without sanctioning any seemingly hostile expressions. We will commit to not be distracted by them and still maintain a professional relationship with them as we help them to process past wounds.

In addition, culturally sensitive supervisory work requires an awareness of diversity and must be able to represent this convincingly in terms of content. Diversity and heterogeneity are an enrichment, they do not make life less complicated, but they do make it richer and more colourful. Not everyone can tolerate this well; those with low self-esteem cannot tolerate much diversity and they may experience diversity as a threat to themselves. In culturally sensitive supervision groups, this can be addressed carefully in the sense of a democratic and identity-stabilising post-socialisation.

Finally, it is important to discover one's own ethnocentric prejudices, to deal with them, to reflect on them and to gain clarity about motivation and biographical experiences. This can strengthen resilient stress and conflict skills with the aim of acquiring 'intimacy and distance tolerance' (Rohr 2003: 513). Because as Waldenfels wrote: 'We can manage to get closer to the stranger when we endure his distance' (Waldenfels, 1997: 179).

Conclusion

Culturally sensitive counselling and supervision is basically and generally the art of dealing with cultural and social uncertainties. These include lack of knowledge, cross-cultural bias, being blind to our own prejudices, and differences in power and hierarchy, differences in the amount of influence they have and their social standing. All of these have an impact on relationships within the supervision group. This requires a self-critical and self-reflective attitude towards oneself—an attitude that allows one to be courageous enough to deal with one's own historical past and the current present from a culturally sensitive perspective. It means not to shy away from, nor ignore or deny, the issues that stand out in terms of cultural sensitivity.

References

Bourdieu P (1986 [1984]) The Forms of Capital. In: Richardson J (ed.), *Handbook of Theory and Research for the Sociology of Education*. Greenwood.

DGSv [Deutsche Gesellschaft für Supervision und Coaching] (2008) *Der Nutzen von Supervision. Verzeichnis von Evaluationen und wissenschaftlichen Arbeiten* [The Benefit of Supervision. List of Evaluations and Scientific Publications]. Kassel University Press.

DGSv [Deutsche Gesellschaft für Supervision und Coaching] (n.d.) Basiswissen [Basic knowledge]. https://www.dgsv.de/beratung/praktische-hinweise/basiswissen/.

Hall ET (1976) *Beyond Culture*. Knopf Doubleday Publishing Group; Anchor Books.

Rohr E (2003) Interkulturelle Kompetenz. Ein gemeinsamer und gegenseitiger Lernprozess in einer sich globalisierenden Welt [Intercultural competence: A joint and mutual learning process in a globalized world]. *Wege zum Menschen*, 55: 8.

Tschetschonig K (2012) *Challenges for Monochronic Individuals in Polychronic Cultures* (English edition; Kindle edition). GRIN Verlag. https://www.grin.com/document/186937.

Waldenfels B (1997) *Topographie des Fremden—Studien zur Phänomenologie des Fremden* [Topography of the Stranger—Studies in the Phenomonology of the Stranger]. Suhrkamp.

Chapter 6

Working with Differences in Mind

An Experience of Group Supervision Training

Marina Gaspodini

Introduction

This chapter focuses on working with differences through the process of supervision—differences in therapeutic orientation amongst the supervisees, their level of experience, their gender, cultural background and class; these differences will reflect and parallel not only the supervisees, including myself as the supervisor, but also the patient population treated by them. This makes for quite a complex tapestry.

These experiences took place during my supervision training to become a supervisor. I was struck by how many differences I was surrounded by and how many levels of complexity the training was trying to address. Within that I became aware of my own difference in relation to others at a personal and professional level. One difference was the colour of my skin: I am White and others were of mixed ethnic background. I am also a group analyst and others were not. I have a level of experience that is different from that of others. I was left wondering how these differences would play out during the supervision training.

In psychotherapy and consequently in the supervision of psychotherapeutic work, there may be a perception that cultural differences have only a relative impact on the internal world of the patient and of the supervisee. However, differences in culture and experiences of racism do have an impact on the internal world of the individual and come into play in the relationship between the patient and the therapist and also between the therapist and the supervisor, and hence the supervision process. Helen Morgan refers to colour blindness 'As a way of avoiding the fear and anxiety which is often present, colour blindness is the denial of differences or its potential consequences. There is nothing to be thought about or to be spoken of' (Morgan, 2008: 7). The knowledge that these differences play a part in the way we relate to others who are different from us allows for an experience of supervision that is far more complex, but closer to the truth of what it is like to be different and still be able to connect to one another. As Helen Morgan says:

DOI: 10.4324/9781032719085-8

What it does do, however, is acknowledge that this is a fact of difference which will impact on the business of getting to know each other. It allows the possibility of the supervisor's unconscious incompetence, and offers the hope that the more paranoid-schizoid links of Love and Hate with racism might be tempered by those of Knowledge. It is not blind to colour but admits an awareness of the political and social backdrop to our encounter with each other. It acknowledges difference in colour and, therefore, a certain difference in experience and hence in vertex or perspective

(Morgan, 2008: 9)

The context of the supervision process

My supervisees were psychotherapists who treated very unwell patients who had needed hospitalisation, including treatment with psychotropic medication. The patients' attendance at their therapy sessions was usually determined by how well they were on the day and, therefore, their attendance at the psychotherapists' groups was not consistent. Furthermore, the therapists did not have a reflective space to talk about the impact of the work and their own group dynamics, which was problematic to say the least. Reflective spaces for clinicians working in mental health are invaluable: the clinicians need to be able to process the impact that the work has on them as well as how they work together as a team. These spaces are needed over and above clinical supervision and line management supervision, and they should be essential spaces rather than impromptu ones. More about this below.

In my earlier training as a psychiatric nurse many years ago, I had the helpful opportunity of working in psychiatric settings not dissimilar from the ones these supervisees were familiar with, and this allowed me to be more in touch with their experiences. Their supervision took place weekly, for one hour, in most of the cases described in this chapter. The supervisees, who sometimes knew each other well, had different levels of experience and training and, as a group analyst, my professional identity and training was different from theirs. There were differences in gender and in culture, male and female and black and brown and white skin colour. The patients they treated were also diverse: a mix of men and women of different ages and social status, with a considerable number of patients of black and brown heritage. This meant different cultures and different attitudes to mental health.

The process of supervision and its complexities

Since the start of supervision, I became aware of the great need that these therapists had for a reflective space, not only for the difficult and challenging work they did but also for their own dynamics as a group. Working in mental health is challenging because we are bound to encounter very tragic stories, people who have suffered through these stories, and intensely painful feelings accompanying them. As mental health professionals, whether a psychiatrist, a nurse or a psychotherapist, we are touched by these stories and we resonate with them. These resonances can be difficult to bear at times. On one hand they help us to empathise with the patient, but on the other hand they may feel too much to bear. Especially in a psychiatric unit or a therapeutic community, the patients' disturbance can be quite intense and their communication often takes place in the form of feelings that are projected onto the staff who must hold those projections and work with them, hopefully to process them and return them in such a way that the patients find them more bearable. However, these projections can feel too much for the staff at times and there may be a wish to return them undigested and therefore unbearable to the patient. These mechanisms take place unconsciously but are detrimental to the mental wellbeing of all involved and detrimental to recovery unless we become aware of them and begin to understand their meaning and function. The latter can be a struggle on a busy ward—for example, where the tasks tend to be medical, practical, concrete, doing things to the patient rather than being with them, determined by pressure to vacate beds, pressure to show 'good' results, or pressure to get rid of 'difficult behaviour'. This is why reflective spaces are essential. They allow the much-needed space to process some of these dynamics, including dynamics between members of staff that, if left unaddressed, make work even more difficult—where, for example, splitting occurs and one member of staff is seen as helpful/good and another as unhelpful/bad. Marcus Evans, in his book about supervision and working in mental health settings, says: 'Patients who split and project are often sensitive to splits in the clinical team as they pick up on rivalries between individual members of staff or disciplines' (Evans, 2016: 52–53). He continues:

> When these feelings get lodged inside, it can make mental health professionals feel guilty or uncomfortable, caught, as they are, between professional ideal of being endlessly tolerant and caring and other negative feelings of irritation, fear, disgust, or even hatred.
>
> (Evans, 2016: 53)

The splitting only exacerbates things between members of staff and staff and patients, if this is not understood in the context of patients' communications and projections, and the patients' need to project. These dynamics, if untreated, lead to staff burnout, illness and eventually departure from the workplace, with consequences for the ward and those left to carry on with the work. It is often thought that staff reflection takes up time away from the work; however, this is a fallacy, and it is more likely to do with a wish to avoid challenging spaces where it is hard to explore difficult feelings and dynamics (in other words, staff reflection needs to take place away from the wards, where it is difficult to explore those feelings). Marcus Evans says:

Patients need to be cared for by staff who are receptive to their experiences and who are willing to take in the patients' communications. In order for this receptive capacity to be sustained in the minds of staff, they, in turn, also need to feel looked after and that senior clinical management take their concerns and feelings seriously. If staff do not feel cared for by management, this affects staff morale, and they tend to become more anxious and less psychologically receptive to their patients.

(Evans, 2016: 41)

I would not have been able to do the work that I did in mental health settings without the presence of these reflective spaces, over and above supervision, which have helped me to process the work I was carrying out on the ward when I was a psychiatric nurse. I remember I used to feel overwhelmed by feelings and by the tragic stories that people shared with me, and I found the reflective practice space fundamental in allowing me to process the level of disturbance present on the wards. Furthermore, these reflective spaces help us to navigate around issues of diversity—cultural, gender and class differences—which play a fundamental part in the struggles that people have with their mental health and that also occur in teams, which are often left unaddressed.

The lack of reflective spaces also makes the task of supervision much harder. Supervision attempts to make sense of the clinical work that we carry out over and above the complex dynamics of team working and the impact that the work has on us as clinicians. When the clinical work takes place in a ward atmosphere where there are difficult unspoken dynamics between staff, these will all play a part in the way we carry out our clinical work. If these issues are not allowed to surface and be voiced and processed, it is very hard to carry out supervision in a meaningful way. This is why the lack of a reflective space for the groups I supervised made my task very challenging.

In a sense, I felt I was in the presence of an almost impossible task that initially felt overwhelming. There was so much to hold. First, the group had to deal with the complexity of the work they carried out with the patients they saw. Then they had to contend with the dynamics of the group itself, with their differences in terms of training, seniority, ethnicity and gender, as well as the previous knowledge of each other in the department, which of course I was not part of. Furthermore, they were also subject to the complexity of the larger dynamics of the hospital they worked for. Finally, and importantly, the complexities of the multicultural (and largely deprived) community they served, which was in a medium-sized town in central Italy, had a direct bearing on their work.

I asked myself whether I was up to the task. Was I good enough for this work? Did I have what it took to take care of this group of supervisees at several parallel levels?

In learning about supervision, I was aware of issues of shame and inadequacy that any supervisor will face at some point or other and with which they will need to wrestle; the training and the reading helped me to be kinder to myself and to learn not to let the harsh voice of the superego dominate. Of course, this is easier said than done, as these dynamics operate unconsciously and it requires continuous and painful work on oneself to become aware of them.

Edward Martin (2005: 172) talks about encountering 'the shadow', drawing on the Jungian concept of the shadow, 'the thing a person has no wish to be' (Driver and Martin, 2005: 172; Jung, 1966: para. 470); and Martin adds 'or, one might add, the thing a person has no wish to know about' (Driver and Martin, 2005: 470). He continues:

> working with the unconscious shadow in supervision therefore carries on the process the supervisee started in their training therapy … constant familiarity with the shadow is essential for ethical therapy—what better place to (re)encounter it than in supervision? But bringing the shadow to conscious thought requires exposure and nakedness and the risk of shame.
>
> (Driver and Martin, 2005: 470)

Of course, the shame in the supervisor mirrors a similar process of facing feelings of shame and inadequacy in the supervisees and this is something that needs to be carefully and sensitively held in mind in the supervision process—to avoid what can be easily experienced as a humiliating process which has the potential to stunt growth instead of facilitating it.

Linked to these ideas around the shadow and feelings of inadequacy was my ability—or difficulties with, I should say—to take up my own authority as a supervisor. No doubt, this would improve with time and experience as well as with continuing to work on being a good enough supervisor. Authority is, of course, an important difference between the supervisees and me, and it is one that carries a lot of weight. Therefore, how authority is used is very important. The idea of owning one's own authority is important in terms of being able to offer the supervisees a space that holds them and their patients, a space that is kind and thoughtful but also one that is robust, where difficult feelings can be contained and thinking is possible, despite the challenges that present themselves.

Jacobs, David and Meyer propose that:

> A basic objective for the supervisor is to promote a safe learning atmo-sphere. Supervision ought to be an enterprise in which the therapist-in-training feels able to think openly, express half-formed ideas, raise questions (no matter how basic), and discuss inner experiences that arise in learning therapy, to the extent that he feels motivated to do so, without undue fear of criticisms, humiliation or intimidation.
>
> (Jacobs et al., 1995: 232)

The supervision training—including the reading—was invaluable in not only helping me navigate my own insecurities but also in helping me understand and appreciate my own capacity to be with others in a genuine and thoughtful way, to attend to what was needed in the moment, to challenge where necessary, and to support and nurture the willingness and ability of others to do the best for their patients. The fact that the supervision training provides supervision of the supervision group, meant that I could take my work to this group and be able to reflect on my own work with the supervisees and to notice parallel processes that occurred in both groups. It allowed for a reflective space in which to grow and develop as a supervisor. It gave me the chance to reflect on what may be going on for me and between me and the supervisees while also helping them to think about their work with the patients. This links back to my previous point about the supervisees needing a reflective space over and above a supervision space and the importance of this.

Experiences of supervision

My experience of supervision is long and varied, from individual psycho-analytic supervision by a kind and thoughtful Jewish man, who used humour to get us through difficult moments, to a videoed mentalisation-based treat-ment group to group analytic supervision, in various different contexts. I was supervised and I have supervised others in all these contexts. The supervision training gave this previous experience structure, learning and collegiality in a way that years of different supervision experience never did.

The training brought all aspects of supervision together, placing them under the microscope to be looked at and considered. For example, whilst I had been aware of boundaries and their importance, to be able to observe and become directly aware of the actual experience of time keeping and time boundaries, of silence and not speaking, and holding these two within a training supervision session, was immensely helpful. Equally, when presenting a clinical situation within a short and strict time boundary, I had felt fru-strated by the shortness of time and therefore I had missed the most impor-tant part of the vignette. In the observer's role, I became aware of what I had missed and where my attention went, as opposed to attending to others' observations, which I had also missed. I found the experience of the super-vision training invaluable in giving me the tools to be present and in the moment in the supervision sessions.

Reflecting on the above learning, made me realise how, in supervision, I cannot take up everything; and what I take up could be determined by something in myself or in the supervisee, or maybe something that happened before the supervision session, or something that may have been in my mind prior to the session. This highlights the importance of one's own awareness and the awareness of others in the supervision process and where the attention goes. This in turn means that lack of awareness of, for example, the importance of differences means that we can be blind to things that are very important in this process.

Differences and intersectionality

Now I want to return to the issue of differences and holding differences in mind. Within the supervision training and the supervision of supervision groups, there was also difference and diversity. One obvious difference was that not all trainees on the supervision training were group analysts; this meant that, in our meetings together, there would be other perspectives. This added to the richness of the discourse, and it required the training organisation to be mindful that the one group analytic perspective did not exclude other perspectives. This paralleled my supervision group where the supervisees were not group analysts. Equally, in my supervision of a supervision group, not all supervisors were group analysts and we all brought different groups in supervision. There were parallels at all levels—training group, supervision group and supervision of supervision group—in terms of the personal and the professional, which run through all groups.

There were other differences, which were to do with skin colour and consequently experiences of racism and White privilege. I was aware that black and brown people were and still are underrepresented in the world of psychotherapy, both as clinicians and as patients, and to me this spoke to the obstacles that there are for these underrepresented groups, obstacles that White privileged people do not have to contend with. They may have to face other obstacles, but they are not faced with prejudice based on skin colour or ethnic diversity.

Furthermore, if we consider issues of intersectionality, whereby other things come to play, such as gender, sexual orientation and class, things can become more complex and the obstacles may be even greater.

Stuart Stevenson speaks movingly and incisively about intersectionality and the position that the group analytic conductor takes when running groups, specifically in relation to analytic neutrality versus positionality. Stevenson challenges the idea of neutrality, and he states that:

> Personal identities relating to phenomena, such as, racism, sexism, classism and homophobia comprise power relational positions rather than just identities based on socially constructed othering. In other words, individuals and groups are embedded within context, systems of power and structural oppression and 'positionality', meaning that our life experiences and circumstances influence how we see and understand the world around us. This understanding is situational, reflecting degrees of privilege, power and oppression.
>
> (Stevenson, 2020: 500)

This of course applies to the position of the supervisor in the supervision group.

The recent events of George Floyd's killing in the United States (and the subsequent movement of Black Lives Matter), the murder of Sarah Everard, and the Me-Too campaign are all issues at the forefront of our minds, the media and the world in general and they can no longer be denied or avoided.

Peggy McIntosh describes White privilege as:

> an invisible weightless knapsack of special provisions, maps, passports, codebooks, visas, clothes, tools and blank checks. ... I began to understand why we are justly seen as oppressive, even when we do not see ourselves that way. I began to count the ways in which I enjoy unearned skin privileges and have been conditioned into oblivion about its existence. I was taught to see racism only in individual acts of meanness, not in invisible systems conferring dominance on my group.
>
> (McIntosh, 1989: 1)

She goes on to make a long list of things that, as White privileged people we totally take for granted.

Guilaine Kinouani talked about Whiteness as an unconscious process that consists of 'a complex multi-dimensional system designed to structure and hierarchize the social thus, the psychological and relational' (Kinouani, 2019: 64).

Audre Lorde, on the point of intersectionality of race and gender, asks 'What does it mean when the tools of a racist patriarchy are used to examine the fruits of that same patriarchy? It means that only the most narrow of parameters of change are possible and allowable (Lorde, 2018: 17). She is talking about changes in women's lives made by those who have an interest in keeping women exactly where they are. The opportunities for changing this are very limited as they are held firmly in the hands of patriarchy, which has very little interest in changing the status quo.

Supervision and difference

Below is a clinical example from a supervision group where clinical issues were discussed and internal group dynamics revealed themselves, including the relationship with the supervisor. This supervision session took place when the supervision group was about nine months old; those present were Sofia, Patrizia and Manuela. Ivano was off sick and Maurizio was on holiday.

Vignette 1: The caretaker supervisor

Patrizia talked about Ivano's group, which she had to cover due to his sickness. While the patients worked using various materials, a particular Black man, Giuliano, talked to Patrizia about the fact that he used to be a bricklayer and plasterer in his country of origin—something that we had not heard before from Giuliano or Ivano. Giuliano had often described the life of abuse he endured when living in an African country and the hard physical work he was forced to do by his extended family, even though he was ostracised by them. It is unclear how Giuliano came to live in Italy except to say that he was tired of this treatment and one day he just left. Since his arrival, Giuliano had been in and out of the psychiatric system and this is how he came to be in Ivano's group. Patrizia talked about Giuliano coming to life when talking to her about his job as a bricklayer and plasterer. Patrizia seemed excited when recounting the story and she wondered with the group what had made Giuliano speak about this. For example, was there a link with Ivano being a White man (as opposed to Patrizia being a Black woman) and was his persecution in his country at the hands of White men; or was it the simple fact that Patrizia was Black that had allowed Giuliano to come to the fore and be seen. Had something in Ivano unconsciously not allowed Giuliano to open up more freely? How was the group, including myself, aware of these internal and internalised dynamics? How easy or difficult was it to talk about them?

I tried to understand both Patrizia's curiosity about Giuliano's disclosure and his need to disclose, considering how difference in skin colour would play a part in this. I asked myself if I had been able to address these issues in the supervision session or had I been reluctant to do so and why?

Supervision of supervision

When I discussed these themes in my supervision of supervision group, I understood Patrizia's struggle and her need for me to get her and get what she was talking about. However, my struggle to respond to Patrizia in a more confident way was perhaps the reflection of a rather paralysing fear of saying something that might offend, which might then reveal my own internalised racism—my concern seemed to be with my own self-image and being seen as racist rather than be up for not knowing, being curious and learning from each other.

What I became aware of was that I was the only White person in the supervision of supervision group (the other White colleague was not present on that occasion). This seemed to parallel Patrizia's position in the group earlier that week. I did experience feelings of being different (as not understanding what is like to be Black), of being stupid, less than the others, and at one point I felt paranoid that my colleagues were picking holes in my presentation. I had a sense, I think, of what it is like to be different, 'of being othered'. It was like a sick feeling in my stomach, and then a wish to disappear and not be there.

However, my supervision of supervision group—including the supervisor—helped me appreciate that I do not have to have the answers, but that I need to be prepared to ask the questions. I did not have to know what it was like to be Black but rather be curious about what it was like for Patrizia to be the only Black therapist in that room with me and the others, on that occasion. My group and the supervisor also helped me to explore those issues and dilemmas, in what was a gentle, thoughtful and kind way.

That session was rather powerful and difficult but a turning point in relation to the sense of feeling not good enough and needing to have the answers.

My supervision of supervision group had richness in it—we all presented very different groups. There was someone who worked in a prison, someone else who brought in work by very young individual counsellors and there was richness and diversity in the presentation of groups from another continent. Therefore, we all brought varied and complex presentations, which were diverse and stimulating, and which added to the learning experience.

The richness that comes in the presence of differences, is an important one because, as group analysts, we value the importance of different perspectives in a group. This sophisticated level of reflection can only occur if there is a structure that allows for that to take place—by this I mean that the supervision training taught me that you do not only need the willingness to explore and investigate your own work as a clinician and a supervisor but you also need these structures to be present and made available to clinicians, like supervision and supervision of supervision. It is only when these structures become *part* of the work—and not an added-on, extra bit—that a true exploration of what goes on between each other and within oneself can take place. This is what the supervision training can allow us to do, and this also applies to the much-needed presence of reflective spaces in clinical settings, as discussed above.

Vignette 2: Marcella

In a different supervision group, which I run online with two supervisees, Antonio and Marcella, we were discussing a female patient of mixed heritage.

The patient was half Eastern European and half Italian, and she was struggling with her allocated nurse who was a White Italian male. It felt as if Marcella wanted to rescue her patient and had become part of this triangle with the nurse; but also, at another level, she may have wanted to rescue her patient from being female and from the tiring task of having to be constantly vigilant about issues of sexism and misogyny being missed. It felt like Marcella wanted to save her patient and offer her a different experience.

As the group became more engaged in understanding the difficulties the patient was experiencing with the male nurse, and Marcella with her, Marcella became less preoccupied with saving the patient and more interested in communicating with the male nurse. Also, she realised she needed to find a way forward for her patient to feel less alone, in the same way that the group was helping Marcella to feel less alone with this patient and to feel less alone with issues of gender and sexuality. As a female therapist born in Italy, I was aware of issues of gender inequality and sexism, and I had to be aware of my own stereotypical views of Italian men and women and make sure that this would not be my own agenda, especially with an Italian male supervisee in the group.

I had to work hard to become aware of my own gender stereotypes and my own history as an Italian woman growing up in that culture while, at the same time, appreciating the struggles of the patient and my supervisees. It was helpful to bring these issues to my supervision of supervision, which I considered a space for me to reflect on my work and my internalised prejudices.

Vignette 3: Manuela

In a different supervision group, Manuela brought a male patient Tarik, with whom she was asked to do some work.

Tarik was from the Middle East, so we discussed issues of intersectionality—ethnicity, gender, and age—as Manuela was not only female but also a much younger person. She had a good grasp of his history of torture and then escape to Italy, and she felt she had established a good rapport with Tarik. However, Manuela became very concerned about the extent of Tarik's trauma versus the shortness of the intervention she was able to offer him. The group were concerned about what it might be like for a man of a different culture, whose body had been violated by torture, to receive therapy from a young female therapist.

As this exploration went on, Manuela became less concerned with what she and her patient may *not* be able to achieve in the little time they had together and more interested in the fact that her psychotherapy would be able to relieve some of the injury to the body and mind of this man, allowing for a possibility of further talking therapy in the future. I was aware of Manuela's young age and that she was doing some challenging work in being exposed to some deep traumatic experiences but had to trust that, despite her young age, she would manage with the help of the group. My wish to protect her in some ways paralleled her wish to protect Tarik from the reality of what we can offer. Both of us had to trust in the capacity to heal even in difficult and limiting circumstances.

It was helpful to make use of the supervision of supervision group, which allowed me to reflect on my wish to protect Manuela, seeing my own younger self in her, as well as on my wish to be protected at times from the challenge of the work we do and what we must face when listening to painful narratives.

Vignette 4: Fostering a supervision group

I was asked to take over a supervision group on behalf of a colleague who needed to take some extended leave at short notice. This group had been meeting online and the supervisees were from different countries, outside the UK.

In a supervision session, Angela brought something quite powerful. It was about a female patient from an African country with whom she had been having difficulties and who had targeted her as a figure of hatred. The patient had become threatening towards Angela. As she explained the situation to the supervision group, Angela became visibly upset—but what was most palpable was her fear. Another supervisee said that the patient had got under Angela's skin, but she had also got under my skin—I felt a pain in the pit of my stomach. At that moment, it did not matter what the skin colour was but that things can get powerfully under our skin. The supervisees became involved in thinking about what could be done—moving into 'doing mode', rather than 'being with' something that felt difficult—like the patient who wanted to do something to Angela.

Was this 'doing to' linked to the fact that Angela was from a country whose people had colonised the African country the patient came from? Angela then told us that such was her fear that she had sought help from management. This 'doing something' seemed to be desperate, but also out of character and not part of the usual protocol. I felt caught up with the supervision group in finding practical solutions, telling Angela to speak to her manager, to speak to the ward. However, eventually, and once the feelings in the pit of my stomach began to lessen, I was finally able to think about what might be happening for the patient and for Angela, and the split between the colonised and subjugated side of both (both frightened) and the powerful and threatening side of both (both frightening). Was this to do with an ancestral and historical conflict between peoples in the colonised African country and the colonising European one?

On reflection, and with supervision, I realised that my White privileged background makes it possible for me to feel able to seek help unlike those who may not have that luxury because of their origins. I reflected on the balance of power given to us by skin colour and position and, in turn, I reflected on my position as the supervisor vis-à-vis the position of my supervisees and how I may be using the power differential in the supervision sessions with them.

The matrix

In the last section of this chapter, I would like to touch briefly on the group analytic concept of the matrix, which was described by SH Foulkes as encompassing the total 'transpersonal processes' of the group, which are affected by communication conscious and unconscious, internal and external, past and present (Foulkes, 1990: 224). According to Foulkes, the matrix includes the personal, the dynamic and the foundation matrices and these are interconnected and not separate, like a web of communication. They communicate with each other and are affected by each other. The social unconscious is part of the matrix; by social unconscious we mean those things that are part of our social and ancestral history, remembered or forgotten, unconsciously or consciously held, and which are part of who we are and who our ancestors were—and therefore inseparable from us. This would imply that issues of diversity, of difference and how these differences are lived, perceived and made sense of, will be part of the matrix of the group. It may be that some of these differences will be in the current discourse of the group, and it may be that others are held in what is yet to be discovered.

The challenge for group analysis is to be meaningfully engaged in thinking and noticing differences while also being immersed in them. The immersion can make us blind to differences, and yet we need to be able both to be immersed and to be standing slightly aside, to observe and appreciate these differences in the group, to notice and feel them, to be aware of them. Maybe this is the paradox of group analysis—being in it and alongside it at the same time, like the matrix that encompasses both the here and now *and* the there and then, both the me *and* the 'thou', at the same time. It is a question of where the lens we look through focuses at any one time. This brings me back to the supervision process as there is a parallel here with the 'third eye' of supervision—the capacity to be in the supervision group with the supervisees and their patients—in a sort of reverie—and then step alongside and observe the interaction—like a clinician with their patient—to provide a supervisory eye, where parallel processes can also be observed and reflected upon.

Conclusion

I have tried to bring alive my experience of supervising psychotherapists while participating in my supervision training, and linking my experience of my supervision group with my supervision of supervision group. I have made working with differences the focus of my writing and, while I have tried to do justice to this topic, I am aware that I have only touched on some of the differences, particularly, though not exclusively, cultural ones. There are many differences when we come to run and supervise our groups and, as group analysts, we value differences because they bring new, 'other' perspectives on what we discuss, which enrich the encounter and push us toward a renewed outlook on the life of the group.

References

Driver C and Martin E (2005) *Supervision and the Analytic Attitude*. Wiley-Blackwell.
Evans M (2016) *Making Room for Madness in Mental Health: The Psychoanalytic Understanding of Psychotic Communication*. Routledge.
Foulkes SH (1990) *Selected Papers of S.H. Foulkes: Psychoanalysis and Group Analysis*. Karnac Books.
Jacobs D, David P and Meyer D (1995) *The Supervisory Encounter: A Guide for Teachers of Psychodynamic Psychotherapy and Psychoanalysis*. Yale University Press.

Jung CG (1966) *The Practice of Psychotherapy.* Routledge.

Kinouani G (2019) Difference, whiteness and the group analytic matrix: An integrated formulation. *Group Analysis*, 53 (1): 60–74.

Lorde A (2018) *The Master's Tools Will Never Dismantle the Master's House.* Penguin Books.

Martin E (2005) The Unconscious in Supervision. In Driver C and Martin E (eds), *Supervision and the Analytic Attitude.* Whurr Publishers, pp. 3–16.

McIntosh P (1989) *White Privilege: Unpacking the Invisible Knapsack.* Wellesley Centers for Women.

Morgan H (2008) The Effects of Difference of 'Race' and Colour in Supervision. *BAPPS Newsletter*: 6–13.

Stevenson S (2020) Psychodynamic, Intersectionality and the Positionality of the Group Analyst: The Tension Between Analytical Neutrality and Intersubjectivity. *Group Analysis*, 53: 498–514.

Chapter 7

EMDR and Art Psychotherapy Group Supervision

Lee Anna Simmons

Introduction

In this chapter I share my thoughts about integrating group analytic supervision with EMDR (eye movement desensitisation and reprocessing) and art psychotherapy supervision.

I start by introducing art psychotherapy and then EMDR (in brief) and follow with a short overview of how I have been combining them. I then detail some of the supervision experience and learning. The reason for my interest in doing this is that I have found art therapy to be a powerful tool for healing, and that, when combined with EMDR, it can reach communities that other therapies might not due to its non-verbal capability of enhancing the ability to heal trauma and attachment wounds across cultures (Holland, 2013).

Supervision is an integral component of professional practice for therapists working with trauma. It provides a structured framework for skill enhancement, ethical practice and the development of a supportive therapeutic environment. Through effective supervision, therapists are better equipped to facilitate healing and foster resilience in their clients. Art therapists often work with the most challenging client groups, those who other services and interventions have given up on: with children and psychosis. EMDR therapists are referred for (complex) trauma cases, hence high-quality supervision is essential for these clinicians. As both an art therapist and EMDR consultant, I find that combining these modalities provides a comprehensive and deeply effective treatment for trauma.

The opportunity to write this chapter has provided a valuable opportunity for me to reflect on the last five years of a supervision group consisting of art therapists who are also EMDR trained: what I have learned, how the field has changed and the next steps. I hope to provide an insight for supervisors of art therapists and EMDR therapists and for the therapists themselves.

Art therapy

'Art therapist' and 'art psychotherapist' are protected titles in the UK, requiring master's-level training and HCPC (Health Care and Professions

DOI: 10.4324/9781032719085-9

Council) registration. There are also music therapists, dance/movement therapists, drama therapists and arts therapists (who combine various art forms in therapy).

The culture of art therapy encompasses various theoretical orientations, with psychodynamic principles playing a significant role. My own training at Goldsmiths University of the Arts, London, reflects a traditional approach rooted in Freudian theory, emphasising rigorous boundaries. In contrast, art therapy training at the University of Hertfordshire leans more towards a Jungian perspective. For instance, dramatherapy at Anglia Ruskin University, London, aligns closely with the Goldsmiths model (which is familiar to me), although supervisees may have attended various art therapy schools across the UK.

Psychodynamic ideas permeate art therapy practice, with concepts such as boundaries, object relations, unconscious processes, projection, counter-transference and transference being central. These theoretical underpinnings inform clinical approaches and interventions.

My academic journey has involved exploring psychodynamic concepts visually, in paintings (e.g., collective unconscious, life/death impulses, trauma healing and envy), drawings (including mapping psychodynamic concepts), live art pieces and social sculptures. Art therapists are expected to be artists themselves, though this can fall by the wayside as clinical work takes over. However, personally I make space for my own art practice and consider it feeds to and from other responsibilities, making it sustainable and, in turn, increasing the sustainability of my clinical practice by offering some protection from vicarious trauma and burnout (Rothschild, 2007).

Vignette: Leon

Leon had been working at a charity using EMDR and art therapy with clients suffering from complicated grief. The members of the supervision group wondered about the impact this might be having on him due to the severity of the cases, which usually involved a terrorist attack, arson, or a stabbing and the underlying trauma for the bereaved. However, Leon was motivated and inspired by helping these clients and had strong boundaries, as well as training in vicarious trauma. Leon made time for his own interests, such as playing drums in a band, spending time with his family, hiking and gardening. When he experienced a bereavement himself, it was similar to one from his early childhood in that it was a shock, avoidable (unfair) and with no time to say goodbye. Leon started to lose interest in his hobbies and to double book sessions and feel relieved when people did not turn up. The supervision group reflected this change back to him and he used his own awareness to take some time to have EMDR himself, after which he moved to a more varied case-load, working at a school one day a week and a hospital two days a week, making time for his family and returning to drumming in the band.

The training in art therapy emphasises group dynamics, offering group supervision, facilitating clinical groups and participating in group art therapy sessions. Trainees also undergo personal therapy, often in a group setting, fostering awareness of institutional dynamics and community functioning. Additionally, art therapists navigate the medical model within mental health settings and address medication-related considerations. Containment, in therapeutic space and time boundaries, confidentiality and consistent studio environments, are all crucial for facilitating client expression and processing unconscious material safely.

Art therapy supports an extremely diverse clientele. Hence supervision encompasses a range of cases, including those that involve refugees, migrants, individuals with eating disorders, victims of child sexual abuse, psychotic patients and clients who have previously resisted conventional therapeutic approaches.

EMDR

EMDR overview

EMDR is a trauma therapy initially developed for use with post-traumatic stress disorder (PTSD) by Francine Shapiro, but is now being used more widely for a range of presentations and clinical diagnoses, working with the body and mind (such as phobias, attachment issues, anxiety and depression; see https://emdrassociation.org.uk/). The training is available to mental health professionals from a range of disciplines. It is taught with a strong framework/protocol, as a basic training to become an EMDR therapist. After a much greater level of experience, EMDR therapists can apply to become accredited EMDR practitioners. The next tier is consultant (accredited supervisor), followed by trainer. This is all part of a system of 'quality control' for EMDR in Europe, the UK and Ireland.

EMDR process

EMDR addresses the distress of traumatic memories through an eight-phase process, integrating bilateral stimulation (BLS) to facilitate the reprocessing of these memories.

The eight phases of EMDR include:

1 **History taking**: The therapist gathers background information, explores past experiences and identifies memories or themes that need attention. A treatment plan/case conceptualisation is created from this foundation.
2 **Preparation**: Coping tools and grounding techniques are introduced so that the process feels safe and manageable. This phase builds trust and ensures readiness.

3   **Assessment**: A specific memory is chosen. An image that represents the event, a negative belief, and a desired positive belief are identified. The level of distress is rated on a scale from 0 to 10 and positive self-belief 1 to 7. Emotions and feelings in the body are also identified.

4   **Desensitisation**: Bilateral stimulation begins (eye movements, taps or sounds). While focusing on the memory, the brain naturally reprocesses it, reducing the emotional charge over time.

5   **Installation**: The positive belief is strengthened, replacing the old negative one. The goal is for the new belief to feel solid and true.

6   **Body scan**: Attention shifts to the body. Any lingering physical tension or discomfort connected to the memory is noticed and processed until calm is restored.

7   **Closure**: Each session ends with grounding techniques to ensure stability. Even if processing is not fully complete, the individual leaves feeling settled and safe.

8   **Re-evaluation**: At the beginning of the next session, progress is reviewed. The therapist checks if previous targets remain neutral and decides what should be addressed next.

Phases 1–3 = preparation, Phases 4–6 = processing, Phases 7–8 = stabilization and checking progress.

This is structured to guide clients from identifying traumatic memories to fully processing and integrating them; it is not always linear but this summary gives the general overview.

In my practice, I use art therapy to enrich each phase, providing clients with a non-verbal, creative outlet to access their unconscious and express their emotions, feelings and experiences.

There have been many new branches to EMDR since its inception in the 1980s. There are additional two-day child and adolescent training and separate accreditation pathways; protocols for addiction and nightmares; and internal family systems. Different parts work with EMDR, and there are many other complimentary approaches to EMDR itself. These include attachment-informed and intergenerational methods developed by Laurell Parnell and Mark Brayne at the Parnell Institute, whereby you can work with experiences as early as being in the womb and trauma wounds of previous generations.

Combining the modalities of art therapy and EMDR

Combining art therapy and EMDR can be achieved by using the following approach that matches the eight stages described above.

• During the history-taking phase, clients create visual timelines, helping to identify and externalise key events.

- In the preparation phase, art therapy techniques like drawing a 'safe place' image aid in establishing safety and trust.
- Assessment involves identifying visual images, negative beliefs and associated emotions and physical sensations, often through symbolic artwork.
- Desensitisation, the core phase of EMDR, employs BLS through eye movements, taps or tones while the client focuses on the traumatic memory. Here, bilateral brushstrokes or drawing (taking the paintbrush, pen or pencil left to right horizontally across the page while following it with the eyes) can enhance the process, engaging both hemispheres of the brain.
- Installation strengthens positive beliefs to replace negative ones, with art activities reinforcing these new cognitions.
- Body scanning to identify residual distress can be supported by body mapping exercises in art therapy, promoting further integration.
- Closure ensures the client returns to equilibrium, often through calming art-making activities.
- Re-evaluation reviews progress, using previous artwork to reflect on changes and reinforce growth.

It is important to note the body scan results and how EMDR is working with memories stored in the body. Somatic expressions are worked with as drawn or spoken words.

The benefits of integrating art therapy with EMDR

Integrating art therapy with EMDR provides a multisensory pathway to healing, enabling clients to access and process traumatic material that may be challenging to articulate. The tangible nature of art products serves as a visual anchor for therapeutic gains, fostering resilience and empowerment.

Personally, I am deeply grateful for the role of art in my life. It has supported me emotionally, provided a means of income, sustained my interest and offered unique ways of exploring the world and our place in it. Art has also served as a form of protest and a medium for sharing information.

The development of my method has been a natural progression, influenced by my diverse professional experiences. My journey began in schools and the social services, where I worked with a wide range of clients, allowing me to understand the varied needs and challenges faced by different individuals. I also undertook a placement in Lebanon, setting up art therapy groups in a refugee camp and addiction service, with the Marion Milner travel bursary from Goldsmiths University (2011–2012). These placements all made me value art therapy and the ability to work across borders and in varied cultures, as well as letting me feel a need to be able to do more—which EMDR helped me navigate.

Transitioning to freelance work and private practice, I established my studio in southeast London, working with self-funders, insurance clients and charities. This setting allowed me to refine my techniques and adapt them to meet the specific needs of my clients. Here I also had the opportunity to combine art therapy and EMDR with children, adapting the techniques to suit younger clients and the educational context.

Through these experiences, I have developed a comprehensive, adaptable method that seamlessly integrates art therapy and EMDR, tailored to meet the unique needs of each client. Prior to setting up the supervision groups I ran training courses and workshops to share these methods, initially with large groups within psychotherapy organisations (the EMDR Association UK and the British Association of Art Therapists) but later in small groups, privately, which unintentionally became a stepping stone to my supervision groups.

Some benefits of group analytic supervision for art therapists using EMDR

In group analytic practice, the dynamic administration (managing clear time boundaries and time sharing) was a part of creating a safe space for our work. We also had time for group discussion at the start and end of each session, facilitating the unpicking of personal narratives and underlying projection and ensuring that countertransference had space to develop along with alliances.

Vignette: using the group to assess a client's need

A supervisee in one of my groups was struggling with one of her clients. Through thoughtful discussion in the supervision group, she was able to think about him holistically and employ her therapeutic training, as he worked through many difficult memories—though not all of them. With input from the supervision group, the supervisee decided that the therapy needed to be much longer-term for her client to work with a memory of finding his father when the father had tried to commit suicide. It can be invaluable to use the group to think about the people we work with, whether they are suitable for therapy at this time, and whether they are suitable for EMDR, because some severely traumatised people dissociate. Groups, with more minds to tune in to what is happening, can be a good place to make sense of it all.

When people have been severely traumatised, listening to their stories can arouse powerful feelings in others. These feelings can be played out within the dynamics of the supervision group. The supervisor needs to be aware of characteristic interpersonal tensions in group therapy as noted by Nitsun. These may be the result of parallel process, taking the form of the dynamics elicited by listening to these traumatic accounts (Nitsun, 1996). Nitsun reminds us that some of the anti-group behaviour that can disrupt a group's task include competition, rivalry, envy, dominance, submission, rejection, group pressure, scapegoating and hostility (Nitsun, 1998).

Vignette: Vickie

Vickie, an EMDR therapist and art psychotherapist, was a member of the Wednesday group for five years. Her feedback at a review was:

> I went to your BAAT (British Association of Arts Therapists) lecture (I think I was mid-way through the Sandy Richman training) and liked your approach. I felt excited by the idea of a group that combined something I was unsure about with something I was more experienced with. It was also a great draw that you understood art psychotherapy and were doing all the leg work of finding ways to integrate the modalities and how they could support and integrate.
>
> Groups are useful places to learn from a rich and diverse source of 'others'—I like to belong to something, and this felt like it would be a safe and nurturing environment to risk and be supported in learning.

Supervision of art therapy

Some years ago, I supervised a group of art therapists working with unaccompanied children, a population facing deeply traumatic experiences with limited resources for therapy. These therapists found techniques from EMDR resourcing—such as safe place, light stream and the four elements—helpful in their work, both with clients and for their own self-care.

To address the potential impact of vicarious trauma and prevent the development of PTSD among these therapists, I implemented group traumatic episode processing (GTEP) during supervision sessions (Simmons and Wright, 2023b; 2023a). This approach allowed supervision group members to process what they had been exposed to and provided a supportive space for reflection and emotional regulation. GTEP uses an A3 sheet of paper with spaces allocated for drawing the safe place, noting the subjective units of distress (SUDS) (levels of disturbance) and placing a symbol or illustration representing the distressing memory. Groups then tap between the past and present dates, following with their eyes with the therapist guiding them, without needing to speak of the experiences (which might be shared or individual to each group member): the levels of distress usually reduce substantially.

Recognising the growing need for art therapists trained in or training in EMDR to receive specialised support, I established a new supervision group that served as a dedicated space for art therapists integrating EMDR into their practice. Here they could receive guidance, share experiences and build resilience in their work with trauma. That was during my time on the

Institute of Group Analysis (IGA) course on group supervision and, as far as we have been able to establish, it was the first EMDR and art therapy supervision group in the world. It seems the training was also inaugural, though the method has increasingly gained traction: in the United States, the book *EMDR and Creative Arts Therapies* was published in 2022 (Davis et al., 2022). This year there was also an EMDR supervision handbook (Logie, 2023) and, in conjunction with *Group Analytic Supervision* (Smith and Gallop, 2023), this has provided the basis for where my supervision framework was situated. Having followed the EMDR consultants training, I was now working with a clinical question about EMDR as well as the psychodynamic base of art therapy. These were in addition to using the group supervision model taught at the Institute of Group Analysis.

Vignette: Paris

Paris turned up flustered and unable to think. She had started a new role in the NHS on an adult ward and had been asked to provide EMDR for a man with a multitude of diagnoses. The group were able to reflect back to Paris that she had taken on some of her client's disorganised thinking and, through this recognition of the countertransference, Paris was able to slow down, re-ground herself and take authority over what intervention was delivered. Paris's client was not a suitable client for EMDR but she could provide art therapy, resourcing and, later on EMDR, once he was more grounded and she had established a therapeutic alliance.

Supervision of EMDR

EMDR supervision is a critical process that enhances the competencies of mental health professionals engaged in trauma therapy. This supervision serves multiple functions, including case review, skill enhancement, ethical oversight and continued education. This is taught to EMDR practitioners who are training to become consultants, to ensure the original eight-phase protocol (Shapiro and Maxfield, 2002) is taught and provides the foundation for the EMDR consultancy meetings.

Supervision sessions typically require a question from each group member relating to a clinical case. Therapists present their experiences, including client responses and therapeutic challenges encountered during EMDR sessions, with the group providing feedback and enabling reflection. The consultant/ conductor holds the group dynamics and supports the experiences of transference and parallel processes as well as eases splitting, scapegoating and other unconscious behaviours that might mirror the client's inner world (and can also arise from the matrix of the supervision group). This is less explored in EMDR supervision (see Logie, 2023) than in art psychotherapy or psychoanalytic supervision; however, supervisors do provide structured feedback, facilitating each therapist's ability to reflect on their practice and adapt techniques as necessary. This reflective process is essential for identifying areas of improvement and reinforcing effective strategies.

A key objective of EMDR supervision is to refine the therapist's proficiency in core EMDR techniques, such as bilateral stimulation and memory processing. Supervisors guide therapists in the application of these methods, ensuring that they are utilised effectively and ethically. This focus on skill development is crucial for fostering therapeutic efficacy and enhancing client outcomes. Supervisors (EMDR consultants) work to ensure that therapists maintain a high level of professionalism, safeguarding the therapeutic alliance and prioritising client safety. This ethical oversight is vital in managing the complexities inherent in trauma therapy, where sensitivity and care are paramount. As EMDR supervision is committed to ongoing professional development, supervisors keep therapists informed about the latest research, training opportunities, emerging practices and advancements in the field of therapy. This is important for maintaining clinical competence and adapting to the evolving landscape of EMDR and trauma treatment. EMDR supervisors are formally categorised as consultants (who provide consultancy), which removes some legal responsibility that a clinical supervisor would carry for the supervisees' clients. That legal responsibility still remains with the supervisor from the clinician's core modality, so, in art therapy and EMDR supervision, distinctions need to be made and contracts need to be clear. Additionally, though countertransference and projection (as well as blind spots and vulnerabilities) are part of what we work with, our work as therapists encompasses more than this. It is important to be transparent when there is not a good 'fit' between supervisor and supervise, whereby minor aggressions between group members and attacks on the supervisor can be survived, worked with and an alliance strengthened. If they interfere with the clinical work then those relationships are better to end.

Reading about the anti-group helped me to know when it was time to close a group that had become toxic. Also important was my peer supervision group from the IGA. This continued to meet after the course ended, but without the supervisor. My own supervision was important for deciding when and how to let a supervisee know I could no longer work with them, either because it was damaging for me or because I felt unattuned to their methodology.

EMDR and arts therapy supervision groups

When I began integrating EMDR and Art Therapy in 2013, I was aware of only one other practitioner in the USA attempting a similar approach. While some art therapists had trained in EMDR, many left art therapy behind, and those who did attempt integration often struggled to find a cohesive method.

My initial research on combining EMDR with art psychotherapy yielded minimal information, with only one MA thesis from the United States addressing the topic. Despite this, I applied the combined approach to my work with people who hoard in a London Borough's social services, achieving remarkable results. Hoarding poses significant safety risks, such as fire hazards and structural damage, making effective intervention crucial and therefore the work was positioned under a safeguarding umbrella. While the number of art therapists incorporating EMDR is growing, most are still relatively new to the modality.

Vignette: Sarah

In a review with Sarah, a psychoanalyst and EMDR therapist, on the third supervision group, which is integrative, her feedback was as follows.

The group setting is a valuable place for differing views when newly qualified and also, I believe, when learning the most from others. The supervision is run with a very thoughtful and pastoral approach, which I have greatly appreciated.

The supervision journey can often feel like a persecutory experience—a sense of judgement and exposure. However, through being a compassionate place this supervision has felt very contained and safe.

Initially I had supervision with an experienced EMDR therapist, which was very helpful in starting to use the method and overcoming 'fear of the threshold' as he put it. Wanting to learn in a group context I joined an EMDR supervision group with a psychotherapist in 2014. This group, comprising a CBT therapist, a clinical psychologist, two psychotherapists and myself, has provided a stable and invaluable resource over the last decade. My supervisor's background as an art therapist and social worker has been particularly beneficial in understanding my cases; and the contributions of artwork in therapy as well create a safe group (with boundaries) that can explore psychodynamic concepts while remaining grounded in the EMDR framework. This, and 15 years of supervision with a group analyst who was previously an art therapist, was useful modelling for my own groups.

Once I, (Lee), became an accredited EMDR consultant and an accredited child and adolescent EMDR practitioner, I received permission to sign off on child and adolescent cases. This led to many newly qualified art therapists and child and adolescent psychotherapists seeking supervision. Initially, managing these requests felt quite messy, but I established boundaries and implemented a process requiring new members to attend individual sessions with me. This ensured they were up to speed with EMDR and were suitable for the supervision groups, rather than the less committed drop-in and ad hoc consultation sessions that work for many EMDR therapists/consultants, but do not work so well for me.

EMDR supervision is based on the protocol that originates with Francine Shapiro. Combining EMDR and art therapy supervision adheres to this also but uses various creative methods in all eight phases.

Vignette: Ramone

Ramone provided EMDR in a prison and had a number of clients he worked with. He used bilateral brushstrokes and other forms of bilateral stimulation (such as the butterfly hug, where the arms are crossed over the chest to make the shape of a butterfly as a form of self-soothing). Bilateral stimulation, a technique from EMDR, has been helpful to prisoners, even though prisoners have not been seen as suitable for the full EMDR approach. People who have not been through all eight phases of the protocol cannot be considered for EMDR—for example, if a client disengages or the therapist realises it is not the right course of action and can explain why.

Art therapists can work with a wide range of clients, and their ability to integrate non-verbal communication through art enhances the effectiveness of EMDR. The artwork can provide a direct route to expressing trauma, which, while healing, also exposes therapists to potentially distressing materials. Therefore, it is essential that art therapists using EMDR have excellent supervision, support in adapting the adaptive information processing (AIP) model and EMDR protocols to their practices, and strong community connections to mitigate isolation. Art therapists often come from arts backgrounds rather than psychology, and may initially need extra support with report writing, statistics and hierarchical structures. Nonetheless, their unique skills and perspectives enrich EMDR practice, offering profound relief and healing to clients. The integration of these two modalities continues to be a powerful tool in addressing complex traumas and fostering resilience.

The influence of trauma on culture in EMDR and art therapy supervision

Culture is the shared fabric of beliefs, practices and values that binds a community. Trauma, when experienced collectively or repeatedly within a society, can alter this fabric, infusing it with a sense of vulnerability or resilience, or both. For art therapists, understanding this interplay is crucial as it informs our approach to treatment and supervision.

Working with trauma survivors, art therapists often become keenly aware of how cultural contexts influence the therapeutic process. The individuals and groups we work with bring their cultural narratives into the therapeutic space, which can either facilitate healing or compound their sense of isolation.

In our supervision groups, the impact of trauma on culture becomes even more evident. The collective trauma experienced by clients can resonate within the supervisory team, influencing our interactions and approaches. A supportive and culturally aware supervision group can mitigate the secondary trauma experienced by therapists, fostering a more resilient and effective therapeutic community.

One of the critical insights from our work is that most individuals would cope with trauma more effectively if they were part of a supportive culture rather than an atomised one. The seclusion and fragmentation characteristic of modern society exacerbate the effects of trauma, necessitating the very services we provide. A culture that emphasises community support, inclusivity and mutual aid can act as a buffer against the damaging effects of trauma.

Community support serves as a powerful preventive measure against the long-term damage of trauma. When individuals feel connected, supported and understood within their communities, they are more likely to develop resilience and coping mechanisms. EMDR utilises 'parts work' (the integration of split-off parts of the self) and also providing clients with mentors and internal safe places where the teams can reside in the psychological inner world of the patient/client.

Art therapy can play a pivotal role in fostering connections in group work, providing a space for expression and communal healing and supporting the resourcing work of EMDR—for example, drawing and 'tapping in' or instal-ling the teams as internal mentors, painting the safe place with bilateral brushstrokes and mapping the support structure of the matrix of the clients, helping them to see the network they are part of.

The powerful effects of culture and trauma and the connections, resilience and sense of containment gained from being in a group are what makes pro-viding group supervision so important when art and EMDR practitioners are working with traumatised people. A typical example of this was given in some feedback by one of my supervisees, Chloe, who was able to put her experience of group supervision into words and has agreed that I can share them here.

> I am struck, that quite often the role of Psychotherapy, can at times, feel an isolated experience. Group supervision provides the pillars of safety and containment to express this without it feeling scrutinised. I have witnessed how the group space can collectively accommodate a mixture of emotions, including a sense of camaraderie. As clinicians, we can often become sub-merged in a client's internal world. However, [it] is the support of other group participants that allows the work to be held and contained in another dimension. This permits the therapist to consider how they are feeling within the therapeutic space and, most importantly, can allow the work to breathe.

Conclusion

Art therapists can often find themselves on the periphery of the therapeutic world, taking on work that others might shy away from or have given up on. Despite not always receiving due recognition for their clinical work, art therapists play a crucial role due to the unique nature of their interventions. Their ability to work both verbally and non-verbally allows them to address issues originating from pre-verbal stages of development, which are often overlooked in traditional, speech-centric therapies. In Western culture, there is a tendency to privilege cerebral and verbal processes, yet the ability to transcend language and cultural divides through image-making proves invaluable. Art therapy enables the expression of experiences too dreadful to articulate verbally, fostering healing across diverse cultural backgrounds. This approach not only challenges the prevailing culture within the therapeutic community but also reshapes it. As art therapists increasingly integrate practices like EMDR, they continue to push the boundaries of traditional therapeutic paradigms, enriching the cultural landscape of mental health care.

Understanding the interplay between trauma and culture is essential for EMDR and arts therapists. Our work not only addresses the individual symptoms of trauma but also engages with the broader cultural context that shapes these experiences. By fostering supportive, culturally aware environments both within our therapeutic practices and in the wider community, we can help mitigate the effects of trauma and promote healing on a collective scale.

Desensitisation and reprocessing painful memories in EMDR successfully necessitates (guided) free association to a client's earliest memories, as a later trauma might have a feeder memory of a similar kind that can stop the processing reaching completion. Hence intergenerational EMDR can involve processing experiences of previous generations—including grandparents—within the inner world of a client, via inherited memories and the internalised ideas of these family figures. This usually results in softer feelings towards the figure/matrix and therefore oneself, often enabling forgiveness on a cellular, deeply felt and somatic level as well as intellectually—enabling lasting change.

References

Davis E, Fitzgerald J, Jacobs S and Marchand J (2022) *EMDR and Creative Arts Therapies*. Routledge.

Holland EB (2013) *Integrating Art Therapy and Eye Movement Desensitization and Reprocessing to Treat Post Traumatic Stress*. Loyola Marymount University.

Logie R (2023) *EMDR Supervision: A Handbook*. Routledge.

Nitsun M (1996) *The Concept of the Anti-Group*. Routledge.

Nitsun M (1998) The Anti-Group: Destructive and Creative Forces in Groups. *Mikbatz: The Israel Journal of Group Psychotherapy*, 4: I–XVIII.

Rothschild B (2007) Help for the Helper: The Psychophysiology of Compassion Fatigue and Vicarious Trauma. *Journal of Psychosomatic Research*, 62.

Shapiro F and Maxfield L (2002) Eye Movement Desensitization and Reprocessing (EMDR): Information Processing in the Treatment of Trauma. *Journal of Clinical Psychology*, 58 (8): 933–946.

Simmons LA and Wright O (2023a) Resources to Support EMDR Therapists' Self-Care. *EMDR Therapy Quarterly*. (Autumn).

Simmons LA and Wright O (2023b) Vicarious Trauma, Compassion Fatigue and Burnout: Tools for EMDR Therapists. *EMDR Therapy Quarterly*. (Autumn).

Smith M and Gallop M (2023) *Group Analytic Supervision*. Routledge.

Part 3

Training and Group Supervision

Chapter 8

Warp and Weft

A Free-Flowing Discussion-Based Model of Group-Analytic Supervision for Psychotherapy Trainees

Joanna Skowronska

Introduction

Grounding the work of a supervision group for trainee psychotherapists or future supervisors primarily in free-flowing discussions fosters their learning of psychotherapy/supervision and their further development of professional skills. When group members communicate with each other in a free-flowing manner, a fabric of relationships, interactions, associations and thoughts is created, referred to by Foulkes as the group matrix (Foulkes, 1990: 154). He believed that this new form of being together is real enough and emotionally lively enough to be meaningful for each participant and yet symbolic enough to be observed and discussed. Therefore, it is potentially able to transform old, non-adaptive relational and mental patterns. In the supervision, the supervision group culture gets imprinted as a new relational network: a relational pattern related to professional practice.

The group-analytic technique is a celebration of collaboration, encouraging participants to engage with each other while simultaneously observing and reflecting on their interactions. As Malcolm Pines put it so well: 'The shared history of the interpersonal relationships in the group and the collaborative effort in deriving meaning from their work together establishes this dynamic group matrix' (Harwood and Pines, 1998; Roberts et al., 1994).

Weaving the matrix

This type of work is akin to the art of weaving fabric. Just as we need a warp, the strands through which the weft is woven, supervisors may find it helpful to keep this metaphor of the warp and weft in their minds to guide their work. It could help them remain sensitive to the necessity of attending to two equally important, intertwined processes that comprise the supervision process and two different aspects of their role.

DOI: 10.4324/9781032719085-11

The warp

Group-analytic supervision group is first and foremost a group. As such it is the scene of all specific group transpersonal processes, which can be viewed as the tacit background and the learning tool. The warp of the supervision group matrix consists of all the activities and processes that promote safety, openness, authenticity and spontaneity. When group participants feel 'held' and 'contained' in a professional situation, the environment can become a 'safe base' for exploring and thinking about themselves, about others and with others. These group processes create a space in which the possibilities for the development of the psychic resources and sensitivity of the participating psychotherapists are multiplied.

The supervisor's roles could be described as those of a convener and a participant as well as a supervisor, applying John Schlapobersky's model of three roles of group conductor to the supervision group (Schlapobersky, 2016). As the convenor, the supervisor plays a key role in ensuring a stable group framework and appropriate group composition. By playing the role of the participant, the situation of professional collaboration is created in which the supervisor's knowledge and experience do not imply any superiority in terms of power or judgement. When a supervisor brings their clinical experience, therapeutic understanding and sensitivity to the discourse, they act as a model for trainees. Their primary task in their role as supervisor is to introduce and encourage a specific type of communication, a free-flowing group discussion, and to help participants navigate it.

A supervision group 'in action'

The following two dreams were recounted in a supervision group for future supervisors.

Dream 1: The dirty nappy

The dreamer dreams that he wakes up because someone is pinching his nose. He opens his eyes and sees that his nose is being pinched by a small boy being held in his father's arms. The dreamer smells an unpleasant smell and suggests that the boy's nappy needs to be changed. But the father says: 'No, that is not necessary.'

Dream 2: Avoiding the precipice

Another dreamer finds himself in a situation where he has to drive and park a car with a trailer attached to the front. In the dream, he feels how difficult it is to drive and manoeuvre this way. He struggles with this task for some time; he manages to turn the wheels of the trailer from the edge of the precipice, and all ends well.

The dreams inspired a group discussion about the psychological situation of future supervisors—people in a transitional phase of their professional development. The challenge of giving up a well-learned skill—conducting psychotherapy—and leaving it to be performed by supervised therapists was discussed.

This problem takes on a particular significance when the supervised therapist is a trainee learning psychotherapy, and the supervision is training supervision. In this uncertain situation, both trainee and supervisor may feel tempted to leave the 'nappy-changing' to those who know better, i.e., the supervisor, and thus disrupt the learning and development of novice therapists.

According to the model of supervision presented in this chapter, the supervisor's task is to allow the supervisee to 'change the nappy' while ideally navigating the work to enable all parties involved to 'park safely'.

The reflections on these dreams alerts the group to the reality of anxieties experienced by all participants of supervision, regardless of their roles. The supervisor's task is to contain both their own and their trainees' anxieties. This is what paying attention to the warp, the part of the fabric that needs to be in place for the group to weave the weft, consists of.

The weft

Parallel to the work on the warp, the weft of the different therapeutic processes is woven into the communicative matrix of the supervision group. The unconscious emotional experiences the therapists bring to supervision are gradually reproduced in the group and reflected in the unconscious emotional experiences of its participants.

> In group-analytic terms, the group supervisees' intra-psychic experience becomes a reflection of the interpersonal and social matrix of the group … In this context, it is as if the training group is, in a transferential sense, re-membered in the here and now of the supervision group—rendering it available, by proxy, to the type of enquiry which is reflection in action.
>
> (Scanlon, 2000: 201)

When the work on the warp of the matrix has been done, the safety and sensitivity of the group participants allow them to search for words and meanings, especially for an experience that has remained nameless, charged with emotions for which no language has yet been found in the therapeutic process, and that 'mumbles to itself secretly hoping to be overheard' (Foulkes and Anthony, 1957/2014: 244).

The supervisor observes the matrix of the supervision group and opens up a conversation and reflection on the work together, helping participants make connections between the therapeutic process that is being discussed and the dynamics of the supervision group.

To grasp the role of the supervisor in weaving the group matrix, it is necessary to understand the importance of the supervisory relationship and the organisation of the training in the case of therapists in training.

Complexity of the role of supervisory relationship in training supervision

All supervision has a two-fold purpose: to catalyse the therapeutic relationship for the benefit of the patient and to enhance the skills and abilities of the therapist. Thus, supervision is an intersubjective field involving three parties: supervisor, supervisee and patient. The relationship between supervisor and supervisee is particularly important in training supervision.

The supervisory relationship is being built on traces of attachment relationships because it serves a similar function. It helps trainees regulate emotions associated with the new professional role and acquire new skills. Through the identification process, the supervisor can serve as a professional role model for trainees and support the development and maturation of their psychological skills such as introspection and reflection, which form the basis underlying all psychotherapeutic work. The safety derived from the contact with the supervisor constitutes the warp of the supervisory relationship. It is vitally dependent on the supervisor's ability to create a safe space. Such experiences can help trainees understand and acknowledge the meaning and nature of therapeutic and supervisory relationships and recognise parallel processes and their intersubjectivity (Stovel and Steinberg, 2008). These are all a part of the supervisor's role in helping their students to form the weft. These two intertwining strands work together to engage epistemic trust: seeking knowledge about the mind and the social environment from those with more knowledge, which is one of the functions of attachment (Fonagy et al., 2017). So, the relationship with the supervisor can become for the therapist in training the foundation for a secure base for professional work, for trust in relationships and in the theories learned, and for their own ability to build on them.

At the beginning of training, however, supervision also implies a student-teacher relationship, with its power, control, hierarchy and dependence issues, contributing to the supervisee's vulnerability. There is, therefore, a fundamental contradiction in the relationship between supervisor and supervisee in training: to fulfil its function, it should be equal, involving the adult, professional self of the supervisee. At the same time, there is an inequality of knowledge and experience, further complicated by the various forms of evaluation inherent in the training. The beginning psychotherapy trainees display a strong need to be guided, to learn about genuinely effective interventions and to earn the supervisor's approval. Furthermore, although supervision is about professional work, it very much involves the supervisee's self and leaves them vulnerable (for example, when their countertransference feelings are discussed).

The role of the context of training

The organisation of the training process also creates problems. Training in psychoanalytical therapies usually consists of teaching theory, the trainee's own psychotherapy and supervision. Ideally, these should coincide in time so that the three processes feed into each other. In the case of training in group analytic therapy, all these processes take place in small groups so that trainees also learn about the importance of group dynamics in action.

> The coordinating of three building blocks of training to proceed in unison aims at imparting meaning and significance to the learning process; it avoids fragmentation and false division between the experience of personal analysis, the supervision and the theory, in this manner facilitating personal growth and authenticity
>
> (Brown, 1995: 25)

The above quote is taken from *The Third Eye*, edited by Meg Sharp, which is based on the experience of the IGA London Group Analytic Training. Therefore, it presents the perspective of a member of the training team. The trainee's experience of the training may be different, especially at the beginning, as illustrated by my dream during my first year of training:

Dream 3: Beginning training dream

The members of the training team are in my flat. They are sitting in my room where they have rearranged the furniture and the books. They are pleased joking and laughing. Although they seem friendly, I don't feel safe or know how to behave.

Beginning training can be pretty disturbing. Psychoanalytic theories are not easy to assimilate at first because they stir the learner's unconscious experiences. Group analytic theory also confronts us with the strength of our connection to others and with the fact that our minds do not belong to us alone.

At the same time, trainees begin their therapy, which inevitably encourages regression. The following quotation from the dream of a person starting training is a good illustration of the anxieties experienced in this period.

Dream 4: A trainee begins their group analysis

> ... he enters the building where his group therapy takes place but has a feeling as though he was about to serve a long jail sentence.
>
> (Hearst and Sharpe, 1991)

Lisel Hearst and Meg Sharpe, citing this dream, suggest that it represents not only the length of time the dreamer has to spend with the group as a part of the training requirements but also his sense that it will take a very long time to correct his 'wrong' personality traits.

Under such psychological conditions, trainees must simultaneously learn how to organise and carry out therapeutic work and, in the case of group analytic training, how to begin to conduct a group of patients. They are required to present their work with patients and to display their inevitable incompetence to their colleagues and the supervisor in the supervision group. They are being persuaded that the process is meant to 'help and support' them. However, the training context, with its various forms of assessment, evaluation and, ultimately, the granting (or not) of professional qualifications, incentivises them to hide rather than to reveal. The supervisor of trainees must be aware of the learners' emotions, able to deal with the anxieties of therapy and supervision in training and able to open a conversation about them. Otherwise, trainees may be tempted to distort the material presented for supervision to fit what they think the supervisor might like. Such lack of honesty casts a shadow on their learning capacity and also on the quality of the psychotherapy they might offer.

Group analytic supervision—a remedy

Group supervision, based on group analytic theory and practice, can be a tool to help trainees overcome the difficulties of beginning training and find a space in which they can enhance the skills and personal resources necessary for psychotherapeutic work. Group supervision is a recognised and valued form because of the specific group factors that create a space that multiplies the learning opportunities. Participants not only receive help with their work but can also learn from discussing the work of others. In addition, the presence of colleagues in a similar position can protect the supervisee's sensitivity and support their *selves* through resonance, mirroring, support and a sense of belonging. Exchanges with other therapists, not only with the supervisor, can be a source of support and foster confidence in one's abilities. The following description of a trainee's experience in a supervision group illustrates this.

My sense of becoming a group therapist began to take shape as my identification with the group and sense of belonging deepened. It brought me a new experience that I was not alone in this developmental process. My ability to focus on the material of other supervisees increased, and I was able to derive more and more satisfaction from helping others. As I felt a sense of connection with my fellow supervisees, I found the feedback they gave me ever more valuable. The way the supervision group was run significantly contributed to my development process. It contributed to my ability to acknowledge my own, sometimes fleeting, insights as essential elements of our shared inquiry.[1]

The trainee therapist absorbs the learning from the supervision group and finds and strengthens their professional *self* within the supervision group process. This student managed to integrate the strands of the warp—the sense of security with the weft—the capacity to learn from the supervision group.

At the same time, the complex interpersonal environment of a supervision group sometimes results in confusion, embarrassment, conflict and rivalry. If these become the subject of discussion and exploration, they have the potential to enrich the participants' perspectives; if not, they can interfere with their professional work.

Vignette 1: The new supervision group

In the newly formed group, participants were very active in giving each other advice and implicit criticism under the guise of analysing the presented material. This created a very unhelpful situation, both for one of the therapists who was struggling with severe problems in her group, no doubt partly related to her personality difficulties, and for the pair of co-therapists who were discussing the patients they had consulted before admitting them to their group and at the same time working on their co-therapeutic alliance.

To be effective, the group must work in a safe and open atmosphere. The supervisor described what she noticed about the flow of the conversation and suggested discussing the reasons behind this. This intervention proved to be fruitful. Discussion of the participants' past learning experiences revealed a harsh, critical object in their minds, ready to judge, chastise and instruct. Identification with this object allowed the group members to avoid falling into the position of someone who was subordinated, criticised and shamed.

This reflection allowed the participants to confront not only the fear of being judged but also the fear of failing to contribute meaningfully to the discussion of their colleagues' groups of patients. Similar experiences at different stages of education, traumatic events, memories of boredom and the lack of a creative atmosphere made everyone (including the supervisor) more sensitive to the presence of this internal object and motivated them to look for different ways of working together as a group.

The example shows how the supervisor intervened in the group's ineffective communication and encouraged the participants to talk openly about it. He was able to do so because he had suggested to the participants that group communication should be based on a group analytic technique: free-flowing group discussion.

Free-flowing group discussion is a multi-person process modelled on the two-person process of free association and the evenly suspended attention of the therapist, as in psychoanalysis. The participants' behaviour diverged from the desired way of working in group analytic training. By encouraging participants to talk about the difficulties of engaging in free-flowing discussion, the supervisor not only ensured safety and openness in the supervision group but also helped participants to reflect on their own experience of resistance to openness and associating with others, which hopefully resulted in their increased sensitivity to similar difficulties they might expect in their patient groups. The supervisor also demonstrated a technique for working with such resistance.

At the same time, this discussion familiarised and introduced the group to a supervisory culture of working with a double task: when reflection on the therapeutic work runs parallel to reflection on the work of the supervision group, they fuel each other.

This supervisor's activity reflects a paradigm shift in group analytic supervision. The terms group analytic supervision and supervision group suggest that supervision becomes a process owned by a group, something they do together, and the supervisor's role is to nurture their work. In this example, the supervisor intertwined the warp—having created a safe working relationship—with the weft: he invited the group to reflect on its own process.

Theoretical concepts underpinning the model of warp and weft

Group analytic situation

Group analytic practice is based on the observation that when conditions are created for a group of people that guarantee an optimum balance between security and freedom, a developmentally rich environment is created where qualitatively new forms of experiencing, thinking and behaving can emerge through interaction with others. Foulkes based his practice on the combination of free-flowing group discussion, a group modification of psychoanalytic free association, the therapist's specific attitude (modelled on the psychoanalytic attitude), and the ability to observe and deal with unconscious group dynamics. He called it a group analytic situation: 'as a dynamic field of experience, and as an aggregate of interactive and interdependent factors of personality and circumstance' (Foulkes and Anthony, 1957/2014: 29). What emerges from this is 'as if they were self-generated by the nature of the situation, which to a great extent they are' (Foulkes and Anthony, 1957/2014: 100).

The group analytic supervision technique requires building a supervisory group analytic situation, an emergent space characterised by safety, spontaneity, flexibility and a spirit of freedom and consent from which new possibilities and meanings can emerge.

Foulkes postulated that specific group factors operate in the group analytic situation. These are the natural interpersonal resources inherent in the situation of people being together: exchange with others involving processes of identification and externalisation, mirroring and resonance, socialisation, the experience of support, the development of the ability to communicate with others, and the condenser phenomenon (Foulkes and Anthony, 1957/2014).

This last is related to the specific form of communication proposed by the convenor: free-flowing group discussion. This mode of communication loosens censorship and thus promotes access to the individual and social unconscious.

Group matrix

In this way, a communicative-relational pattern is created called a group matrix (Foulkes, 1964: 5). It manifests itself at different levels, ranging from the most visible, accessible to consciousness, to the more unconscious (Foulkes, 1990: 183).

The first level—the dynamic matrix—results from the mutual experiences, relationships and understanding built up when people talk freely in a group. According to Pines, 'The shared history of the interpersonal relationship in the group and the shared work in deriving meaning from their work together lays down this dynamic group matrix' (Pines, 1998: 68). At this level, the group represents for participants their community or social group. In a well-functioning supervision group, the group culture, characterised by friendliness, inquisitiveness and curiosity about psychological life, impacts the functioning of its participants in professional groups.

The transference, projection and foundation matrix levels feed and influence the dynamic level. The transference level refers to the psychic contents in the group that are related to the transfer of emotions, expectations and attitudes from meaningful life relationships to the group supervisor and members. In particular, the supervisor usually becomes a transference object of desires and fears from parental and authority figures. The projective level concerns the psychic material related to projecting aspects of the self and objects onto the supervisor and reciprocally between group members. In a supervision group, this level may manifest itself in the less experienced member of the group attributing desired mental and emotional qualities to the supervisor and more experienced colleagues, as if to deposit them, thus feeding the illusion that they too will be so wonderfully equipped and unthreatened by uncertainty or error in the future. Conversely, it is the other participants in the group, or a particular participant, who becomes the object of projecting undesirable aspects of professional attitudes so that the person projecting can feel free of them and not work on them.

According to Foulkes, the foundation matrix level is the common ground, partly biological and partly social. What is essential in supervision is that it is the level at which we collectively know or do not know certain things. It gives rise to certain shared, non-negotiable attitudes directly assimilated through generations. The foundation matrix influences the other manifestations of the group matrix. It may result in the therapist's ignorance of certain aspects of the patient's experience, such as ethnicity, class, gender, disability and others. Access to this level via supervision depends mainly on the openness and social sensitivity of the supervisor. At the same time, in a supervision group, as in any group, this area is a 'condenser' of metaphors and images and a source of associations.

The group analytic technique generally allows all matrix levels to become objects of interaction, conversation, reflection and repair in the dynamic matrix.

When the supervisor is working with the weft, they observe the manifestations of the matrix levels and open up a conversation and reflection on the work together, helping participants make connections between the therapeutic process being discussed and the dynamics of the supervision group (Pines, 1985: 27).

Free-flowing group discussion in the supervision of trainees

Therapeutic craft involves knowledge, technical skills and the therapist's accumulated experience. The last combines the therapist's personality, sensitivity and relational experience with the patient.

In dynamic psychotherapy, at least two types of knowledge, representation and memory, are engaged and reorganised. One is explicit (declarative) and the other is implicit (procedural) (Stern et al., 1998).

The 'declarative' aspect is overt and accessible to consciousness. It can be expressed symbolically, in images, or verbally. In this area, the transformation from unconscious to conscious takes place through interpretation. Supervision based on the 'declarative' aspect concerns knowledge and understanding. Procedural knowledge of relationships, on the other hand, is implicit and operates outside the conscious experience available for verbal elaboration. The 'unthought-known' (Bollas, 1987) and Bowlby's 'internal working models' (Bowlby, 1969), or Stern's 'ways of being with another' and 'implicit relational knowing' (Stern, 2018; Ellman and Moskowitz, 2008) are examples of how different authors tried to capture this non-symbolically represented dimension.

According to researchers from the Boston Change Process Study Group (BCPSG, 2010) the change achieved in psychotherapy depends significantly on the work in this area (Ellman and Moskowitz, 2008).

The supervision of psychotherapies, especially psychodynamic ones, requires access to this area and the ability to master ways to develop the necessary skills. Christopher Scanlon distinguishes between two types of reflection we need in supervision: reflection *on* action and reflection *in* action. Reflection on action occurs when we consciously reflect on the process of psychotherapy. It is based on consciously remembered material and refers to theoretical concepts. Although it allows hypotheses to be formulated about the unconscious in the therapeutic encounter, it does not provide access to the unconscious experience of the therapist and patient. It refers to what the therapist knows and can say and leaves out what the therapist does not know and cannot say. It does not touch the internal, unconscious, limitations of the therapist. According to Scanlon, supervision based only on this type of reflection is of limited relevance to the therapist's professional development. Reflection in action, on the other hand, requires enduring uncertainty and a lack of clear understanding of what is happening, waiting for a more 'meaningful figure' to emerge. It requires focusing on the here and now of the supervision session to allow access to the therapist's knowledge derived from encountering another person—the patient (Scanlon, 2000).

Free-flowing group discussion is a vehicle for interweaving more conscious, unconscious and implicit aspects of the psyche. This kind of communication allows all the specific group processes of mirroring and resonance to go on in the background, all the while enhancing the process of teaching psychotherapy, as they create a space that fosters the development of the psychic resources of participating psychotherapists.

In the supervision group, the ability to maintain this kind of exchange with others is the therapist's 'Ego training in action' (Foulkes, 1990: 181), the exercise consisting of honing professional skills while retaining the capacity for self-observation. The indirectness, freedom and democracy of association allow the supervision group to act as a catalyst in which the unconscious content of the supervised therapeutic processes, intertwined with the unconsciousness of the participants in the supervision group, is amplified and can become the object of interpersonal exchange, thereby opening access to previously unconscious experiences that were impossible to articulate.

Let us take a look at another supervision group 'in action'.

Vignette 2: The unexpected break

In the following example, the supervisor helps the group to weave the weft by addressing their resistance to getting engaged in communication about their work.

A therapist whose patient group had been running for two years and was coming to an end, with only three months left, unexpectedly took a few days off and missed a supervision session. His difficulties in facilitating open communication in the group had been discussed previously. The therapist returned full of energy for the following session and apologised for his absence, saying he needed a rest. He was the first one to submit material from his group. Presenting a transcript of the session, he emphasised with satisfaction that his patients had talked a lot about how beneficial their therapy was for them. With obvious irritation, he spoke of a patient who did not match the group's mood, relentlessly voicing depressive thoughts.

After he finished the supervision group kept silent for quite a while. The supervisor commented that such prolonged silences were unusual for this group.

Someone said that she was holding back because the therapist seemed hurt. This participant added that although she had experienced the benefits of attending the supervision group, there were times when she felt hurt when her point of view or what she was experiencing was not understood. Others added that patients in the group were likely to be anxious about the imminent end of therapy. They pointed to moments in the material that triggered such associations in them.

In response to these group associations, the presenting therapist cited a dream of one of his patients: the patient had dreamt that an explosion had blown up the Palace of Culture and Science,[2] exposing the ground underneath. Injured and mutilated people came out of dungeons. The dream provoked a lively resonance. Someone mentioned that the Palace had been built on the site of the former ghetto; someone else recalled that a number of workers had died during the construction of this monumental building. Someone else remarked that the people who came out of the underground were injured yet alive.

Further discussion on the exchanges in the supervision group helped participants reflect on the possible feelings of the group of patients. Supervisees were talking about past traumas, making separation difficult for the next generation, equating it with a catastrophe. There was discussion about possibly explosive feelings arising from the therapist and the group apparently 'building the Palace of Culture and Science' together. The people in the dream, like in the group, were alive; but, by celebrating a false success, they may miss the opportunity for a new beginning – one that might be less spectacular than the Palace of Culture and Science but would give them access to a living experience rather than a dead one. Everyone, including the therapist presenting the material, was deeply moved.

The theme of false success as a defence against the experience of uncertainty and loss prompted another person to come forward and share her dilemma.

We can see how a rupture in the matrix of the patient group, recorded in its therapist's experience, is played out and then read out in the supervision group. It became possible to see the total situation related to the therapist's previously discussed difficulties in deepening the group discussion. The therapist's problem could be understood and worked through as a disturbance in the relational network at all levels of the matrix of his group.

In the vignette above, we see a reasonably mature supervision group, meeting regularly for about two years, on a fixed schedule, for a fixed amount of time, and whose task it is to discuss therapeutic processes in the group conducted by its participants. It is large enough to offer a wealth of viewpoints and sensitivities yet small enough that at each meeting all participants have a chance to present material from their group and be engaged and active. The group's members are at different stages of training, with varying levels of therapeutic experience and various lengths of participation in the group. Such group composition allows newer participants to build on the experience of older ones who have already experienced the difficulties and anxieties of starting training. The enactment described in the vignette could take place because the participants have had several experiences in which they have felt free to reveal their difficulties without being too ashamed of themselves. As in the above example, the experienced discomfort has been rewarded by removing blockages in the experience of the therapist and the group. It is not uncommon for the therapist to come to the next meeting after such an event and say, 'My group talked as if they had been with us in the previous supervision'.

We can observe how, through the mirroring of the presenting therapist's feelings (a participant who speaks of his vulnerability to being misunderstood) and the feelings of the patient group members (resonance with the fear of the impending end), the participants in the supervision group and the presenting therapist gain insight into the risk of not recognising the painful feelings present in the therapy group associated with the impending end, hidden under the defensive veneer of the proclaimed benefits of psychotherapy. The supervisor's intervention in the form of a comment on the unusual behaviour of the supervision group proved sufficient for the group to overcome the blockage in communication, and a process of free-flowing group discussion, and thus a process of translation of the unconscious into available consciousness, took place.

Parallel process in groups

The interweaving of the matrices of the supervision group and the therapeutic groups is the group equivalent of the phenomenon described as a parallel process in supervision. Margaret Smith and Margaret Gallop propose the following model for working with the interweaving of the matrices of the supervision group and the matrices of the therapeutic relationship being supervised.

The six-step model for working with the parallel process in the supervision group:

1   Encourage each member of the supervision group to be an active 'third ear', i.e. sensitive to emotional pushes and pulls and group dynamics (Billow, 2011).
2   Acknowledge that a parallel process has taken place.
3   Tolerate and contain uncomfortable feelings.
4   Restore emotional balance.
5   Reflect on the experience in the group in a non-defensive way.
6   Ensure that the supervisee who has presented their work has been able to hear what has been said in a way that is helpful for their work (Smith and Gallop, 2023: 179).

In Vignette 2 above, we see the participants in the mature supervision group making connections between their associations and the emotions they evoke, as well as the experiences of the participants in the patient group. The supervisee's retelling of the patient's dream about the explosion that blew up the Palace of Culture and Science, through the meanings shared in the foundation matrix of the supervision group, opens access to reflection on the emotional experience of the patient group. A supervisee's comment about people coming out of the dungeons alive translates meanings arrested in the past into the language of the present experience of people in therapy. It is a good example of the condenser phenomenon described by Foulkes:

> The term condenser phenomena is used to describe the sudden discharge of deep and primitive material following the pooling of associated ideas in the group. The interactions of members loosen up group resistance, and there is an accumulative activation at the deepest levels. It is as if 'the collective unconscious' acted as a condenser covertly storing up emotional charges generated by the group, and discharging them under the stimulus of some shared group event.
>
> (Foulkes and Anthony, 1957: 199)

Through the interplay of reflection in action and reflection on action, the grandiose, false self is confronted with the *true self* developed in therapy. Now, fragile and vulnerable, moved by the prospect of impending separation due to the completion of treatment. Having achieved this level of sensitivity, the group conductor can accompany the participants in further growth. In this established supervision group, the participants have developed their capacity to work with the weft, connecting with what had been unconscious through their free-floating discussion and ability to use images that capture the unconscious content of the material.

Two models of introducing free-flowing group discussion into supervision in groups

Foulkes recommended that when introducing free-flowing group discussion, the principle of minimum instruction should be maintained (Foulkes, 1948). We cannot do the same in a supervision group if we want it to fulfil its primary task. I now present two models of supervision group organisation I rely on in my practice.

Model of group reverie[3]

In their supervision group model, the authors Avi Berman and Miriam Berger rely on a combination of Foulkes' concept of the group matrix and Bion's *reverie*. (See Berman and Berger (2007) for a detailed description of this model.) Group participants are encouraged to listen to the material presented in the following way:

- Be yourself when listening to the presented material.
- Pay attention to your inner world: feelings, emotions, fantasies, memories, thoughts.
- Take your time, listen to yourself.
- Share what emerged in you while you were listening.
- Free yourself from the compulsion to praise or criticise.

(Berman and Berger, 2007: 244)

According to Berman and Berger supervisors should ensure that group members do not ask the supervisee questions about the material presented and refrain from making personal or professional references to the supervisee or their patients (common and acceptable ways of relating to the content presented for supervision). Instead, we invite participants to turn their attention inward and listen to themselves. They can share with the group anything that emerges from their *reverie*. Sharing it marks the transformation of the private into the social sphere and naturally creates emotional tension that can accompany participants as they get in touch with the patient's and/or therapist's painful feelings. The experience of mirroring in the professional situation, of accompanying the relationship with the patient(s) 'brings the supervisee back from the emotional exile to which they may have felt condemned when he struggles with his professional difficulties alone' (Berman and Berger, 2007: 245). It strengthens their ability to accommodate the patient's feelings and develop confidence in their resources.

Berman and Berger propose that the group move on to more task-focused work after the initial free-associative part. At the end of each presentation, the presenter has time for reflection. In beginner groups, I ensure that the session is structured in this way; this rhythm becomes second nature for more mature groups.

Vignette 3: The supervision group reflects on its process

A beginner therapist presented the material from her newly started group of young adults. She cited mature and wise exchanges between participants and her apt interventions. The participants in the supervision group, including the supervisor, were very impressed. They plunged into a lively intellectual, theoretical discussion. Then one participant said: 'Wait a minute, let us stop; we forgot our associative work!' The supervision group mirrored the patient group's communication matrix and only upon reflecting on the reasons for such communication were they able to uncover the emotional content hidden under all this sophistication.

In the above vignette, we can see how the intellectualisation and emotional isolation evident in the patient group were replicated in the supervision group. The group, alerted by the comment of an attentive member, were able, through free group discussion, to understand that the latent desire to gain recognition and attention from the therapist in the patient group, which may be natural in the initial stages of therapeutic group development, was compounded by the somewhat distanced and intellectual style of the therapist vying for the recognition of the supervisor and the supervision group. In this way, a thread is woven into the warp of the matrix of the supervision group: participants get an understanding of the experiences in the therapeutic group by connecting them with theirs, which becomes the pattern of their work with the patients' group.

The persistent groundwork laid by the supervisor in helping this group of therapists to work with the weft had allowed one of the people in the group to stand back and reflect on the group process. In this example, the task of moving from reflection on action to reflection in action is now a task of the group rather than the responsibility of the supervisor.

In a well-functioning supervision group, supervisees' resonance with colleagues' work can be a resource, and their free associations have the potential to deepen their understanding. At the same time, we can see how the supervision group reproduces unconscious dynamics from therapy and needs a 'third eye' to recognise the parallel process. In the case described, this role was fulfilled by an attentive group participant.

Model of group supervision using a reflective team

The model of group supervision using a reflective team was developed for the Diploma in Supervision training at IGA London and is written about in more detail in a paper by Smith (Smith, 2019). It is summarised here in brief to illustrate its use with supervisors involved with training students. Organising the supervision group meeting in this way creates an experiential learning situation about the importance of working with countertransference, resonance and parallel processes in group supervision. The multiplicity of perspectives in the intergroup space of supervision with a reflective team fosters the development of a 'negative capacity'—the ability to endure a not-knowing stance and maintain a state of curiosity.

The supervision group is divided into two subgroups. One of them works on the therapist's problem presented for supervision. The participant in this subgroup takes on the convenor role, and their task is to take care of the group's time boundaries and free discussion. Another subgroup constitutes a reflective team similar to the one used in family therapy. The team observes the group conducting the supervision and then shares their observations about the observed conversation. The two groups then discuss their experience in a free-flowing group discussion, relating it to the problem presented.

An important aspect of this model is how the supervision material is presented. The presentation should be brief—a 'snapshot'—and include an exchange with the patient or group that has affected the therapist's ability to think and react at the time—an indicator of a countertransference response.

This way of working allows group participants to deepen their ability to work with countertransference. It teaches the therapist to distinguish between resonance and the aspect of countertransference that diminishes the therapist's ability to reflect on the therapeutic relationship. Unrecognised, countertransference leads the therapist to under- or overidentify with the patient, which can block the effectiveness of therapy. It is easier for the therapist to recognise their weaknesses when they find them in the associations and reactions of colleagues than when the same feedback comes from the supervisor from their position of expertise.

The supervisor's task in this experience relays on creating a climate of trust and familiarising the participants with the structure of the proposed experience. They need to ensure that participants share their feelings, experiences and points of view, rather than suggestions and questions, to reduce the fear of exposure and embarrassment in the supervisee presenting their work.

In the final part, when the parallel process is recognised, the supervisor's task is to help the group members use the experience to gain insight into the therapeutic relationship.

Vignette 4: Reflecting team supervision

Two co-therapists presented a relatively 'young group' in the supervision group. They were concerned about the group's lack of emotional response to one member's dramatic behaviour after the previous session. They were concerned that the group were unable to engage emotionally withdrawn patients in a more empathetic way.

The reflective team spoke of the high emotional charge they felt in the group. They pointed to the participants' appreciation of being together, as opposed to the abandonment they had experienced in their lives. They pointed out that when one patient extolled the prospect of hospitalisation as a guarantee of not being alone, the disturbed patient seemed to feel understood. One person needed help figuring out the date of the described session, which turned out to be the last one before the scheduled Christmas break.

During the shared conversation, the co-therapists expressed surprise at the emotional resonance of the reflective team and felt relieved. One of them admitted that she had bad associations with the pre-Christmas period and usually simply waits it out as if frozen.

While listening to the reflective team talk, the 'frozen' therapist independently discovered her 'blind spot' preventing her from resonating with the patients' experiences. Such an act of introspection in the supervision group can potentially become a model for reflection in the patient group, as it is not accompanied by embarrassment or other tension-inducing feelings.

Smith's model is also helpful for large supervision groups. All participants are involved, and the situation is more democratic. The presenting therapist is not the only one exposed to group scrutiny, so the embarrassment accompanying the presentation and the dominance of the supervisor as an expert are avoided.

Smith emphasises the importance of basing the conversation in the supervision group on free-flowing discussion, an undirected, non-goal-oriented mode of communication that, as experience shows, encourages the sharing of personal experiences and the emergence of associations and metaphors containing emotions. It is conducive to participants making connections between supervision and psychotherapy situations as opposed to the frequent defensiveness resulting from questioning or insightful inquiry.

In such a situation, the supervisor can put themself more in the position of a group participant and bring their personal and clinical sensitivity into the process of free association. This makes the supervision process more democratic by allowing the participants in the supervision group to develop their free-thinking skills. When all participants in the supervision session function on an equal footing, the supervisee and the supervisor are freed from a position of dependence or unquestioned authority.

The importance of the training institution

Finally, I want to point out the importance of the training institution and relationships within the training team and the relationship of trainees and teachers to the training institution as a whole.

It should not be forgotten that the network of relationships between staff can become a fertile ground for conflict and tension (Hilpert, 1995). Also, any overlap and interaction between the groups involved in training can bring about some fissures. One of the most frequently observed phenomena is the splitting of trainee transference between the individual group therapist and the supervisor or didactic seminar leader. In turn, unresolved conflicts between a supervisor and another member of the training team or the institution where the supervision occurs can lead to the supervisor playing out their conflict with a colleague or institution in a corresponding role reversal with one or more of the supervisees (Kernberg, 2010).

Again, the free-flowing group discussion in the supervision group is the optimal means of opening conversations about institutional conflicts that may affect supervision and other training elements. An unrecognised or unresolved parallel process of countertransference creates a feedback loop for the relationships between supervisor, supervisees and their patients. Such interpersonal and intergroup processes are the natural substrate of all therapeutic work in the broader systems. Supervisees become more sensitive to the importance of the context of their work for the therapeutic relationship.

Talking openly with trainees about the training context can also be beneficial for trainers' professional development. We have all been trainees at some point in our lives, and we have all been supervised in training, which has influenced our attitudes to supervision, formed certain habits, and established ways of working that we may continue without much reflection.

Conclusion

Although supervisors often work with the elements of warp and weft, it can also be useful in working with students as it helps highlight the tension between the supervisor's role as a container and that of an educator. This chapter illustrates how the supervisor might negotiate their roles as a container and an educator and allow the group to take over from them.

Notes

1 Excerpted from a final essay by a participant in a group analytic training course at IGA Warsaw. Included with her permission.
2 The Palace of Culture and Science is a huge building in the centre of Warsaw. It was a gift from the Soviet Union to the Polish people while Poland was under occupation and was intended to alleviate and negate their fear and sense of loss after the invasion of Poland by Germany in the Second World War. However, it still evokes ambivalent feelings in Poles.
3 The model is described in detail in the article Berman, A. and Berger, M. (2007) Matrix and Reverie in Supervision Groups. In Group Analysis 40 (20) 236–250

References

BCPSG (2010) *Change in Psychotherapy: A Unifying Paradigm*. W.W. Norton.
Berman A and Berger M (2007) Special Section: Matrix and Reverie in Supervision Groups. *Group Analysis*, 40 (2): 236–250.
Billow RM (2011) It's All About 'Me': On the Group Leader's Psychology. *Group Analysis*, 44 (3): 296–314.
Bollas C (1987) *The Shadow of the Object: Psychoanalysis of the Unthought Known*. Columbia University Press.
Bowlby J (1969) *Attachment and Loss*. Vol. 1. *Attachment*. Basic Books.
Brown (1995) Simultaneous Supervision and Analysis. In Sharpe M (ed.), *The Third Eye: Supervision of Analytic Groups*. Routledge.
Ellman S and Moskowitz M (2008) A Study of the Boston Change Process Study Group. *Psychoanalytic Dialogues*, 18: 812–837.
Fonagy P, Campbell, C and Bateman, A (2017) Mentalizing, Attachment, and Epistemic Trust in Group Therapy. *International Journal of Group Psychotherapy*, 67: 176–201.
Foulkes SH (1948) *Introduction to Group-Analytic Psychotherapy*. Heinemann.
Foulkes SH (1964) *Therapeutic Group Analysis*. George Allen and Unwin.
Foulkes SH (1990) *Selected Papers of S.H. Foulkes: Psychoanalysis and Group Analysis*. Karnac Books.
Foulkes SH and Anthony EJ (1957) *Group Psychotherapy. The Psychoanalytic Approach*. Penguin.

Foulkes SH and Anthony EJ (1957/2014) *Group Psychotherapy: The Psychoanalytical Approach*. Karnac Books.

Harwood IN and Pines M (1998) *Self Experiences in Group: Intersubjective and Self Psychological Pathways to Human Understanding*. Jessica Kingsley Publishers.

Hearst L and Sharpe M (1991) *Training for and Trainees in Group Analysis*. Tavistock/Routledge.

Hilpert HR (1995) The Place of the Training Group Analyst and the Problem of Personal Group Analysis in Block Training. *Group Analysis*, 28 (3): 301–311.

Kernberg OF (2010) Psychoanalytic Supervision: The Supervisor's Tasks. *The Psychoanalytic Quarterly*, 79 (3): 603–627.

Pines M (1985) Psychic Development and the Group Analytic Situation. *Group* 9 (1): 24–37.

Pines M (1998) *Circular Reflections: Selected Papers on Group Analysis and Psychoanalysis*. Jessica Kingsley Publishers.

Roberts J, Pines M and Shapiro ER (1994) The Practice of Group Analysis. *Journal of the American Psychoanalytic Association*, 42 (3): 955–960.

Scanlon C (2000) The Place of Clinical Supervision in the Training of Group-Analytic Psychotherapists: Towards a Group-Dynamic Model for Professional Education? *Group Analysis*, 33 (2): 193–207.

Schlapobersky J (2016). *From the Couch to the Circle: Group-Analytic Psychotherapy in Practice*. Routledge.

Smith M (2019) Through a Glass Darkly: Using a Reflecting Team Approach in the Development of Supervisory Practice. *Group Analysis*, 52 (3): 297–312.

Smith M and Gallop M (2023) *Group Analytic Supervision*. Routledge.

Stern DN (2018) *The Interpersonal World of the Infant: A View from Psychoanalysis and Developmental Psychology*. Routledge.

Stern DN, Sander LW, Nahum JP, et al. (1998) Non-Interpretive Mechanisms in Psychoanalytic Therapy: The 'Something More' than Interpretation. *The International Journal of Psychoanalysis*, 79 (5): 903–921.

Stovel L and Steinberg P (2008) Learning Within Psychotherapy Supervision. *Smith College Studies in Social Work*, 78: 321–336.

Chapter 9

Cultural Sensitivity and Training for Supervisors of Groups

Margaret Smith

Introduction

The understanding we have about what makes good training is shaped by the values inherent in our culture. When we are working with a multicultural group, as trainers or as supervisors, we need to keep culture in mind. Foulkes understood that culture has a significant impact on shaping each of us. 'The individual in life is equally determined by the various groups of which he is a part, some more, some less fundamental: his culture, his nation, his family, his clan, his time' (Foulkes 1964: 168). The ego and superego have been shaped by identification with others throughout life (Foulkes, 1990: 59). Trainers and students may have different culturally determined expectations about what training is offered, what their role is and how best to deliver training in order for students to learn. Developing sensitivity to cultural norms and differences, the style of delivery and the dynamic administration, and spending time orientating students to the training can make a difference to students' capacity to learn.

Culture and group analysis

The core values of group analytic supervision training come from Foulkes' understanding of the relationship between the individual and society. The social and cultural dimension of a society will shape the experience of all the individuals within it. It is the group, not the individual, that forms the basic psychological unit. As individuals develop, the society they belong to penetrates each person to the core (Foulkes, 1948: 14–15). This chapter explores effective teaching and some of the qualities that contribute to a good learning experience for students. It moves on to address the things that contribute to a culturally sensitive course when teaching a diverse student group. It makes links with culturally sensitive approaches to training and the way the IGA supervision training equips therapists to become supervisors.

DOI: 10.4324/9781032719085-12

The qualities of a good trainer and the methods they use

Marsh and Hattie found that expertise in their field alone did not guarantee the effectiveness of learning by students (Hattie and Marsh, 1996; Marsh and Hattie, 2002). This makes it important for organisations to inform and support trainers in developing skills that contribute to a student's learning (Sierens et al., 2010).

Titsworth found that students were affected by the trainer's level of engagement with the group, picking up non-verbal signals from their body language as well as verbal cues. He found that students learned best when they felt the trainer was friendly and approachable, and actively engaged with the group. This was conveyed through their eye contact, smiling, their use of humour and their tone of voice. Good trainers were experienced at making the student feel closer to the trainer, increasing their engagement. When trainers' input promoted long-term learning, they also summarised the format for their presentation, used personalised examples, and highlighted those things they saw as key aspects of what they were covering (Titsworth, 2001).

However, active trainer participation was not enough on its own. Learning also requires active participation on the part of students. O'Hair, O'Hair and Wooden made a connection between students' effective listening skills during lectures and good academic performance (O'Hair et al., 1988). Sierens found that effective learning also required students to be motivated, have their own goals and a sense of agency. Students learned best when they had a sense of their own autonomy (Sierens et al., 2010).

Trainers enhanced learning when they:

- encouraged students
- engaged well
- listened to students' views
- framed their input in the form of questions and answers
- used examples that supported their application of the material to the real world (O'Hair et al., 1988)
- had a clear lesson structure (Sierens et al., 2010).

The impact of culture on learning

An individual is often blind to many aspects of our culture. 'We are all part of a social network, a nodal point, as it were in this network, and can only artificially be thought about in isolation, like a fish out of water' (Foulkes, 1948). We cannot see the things about our culture that are taken for granted unless we stand outside of it.

Some differences between cultures

In a study of differences in approaches to learning between Eastern and Western cultures, a literature search by Jin Li makes a connection between cultures and their underpinning philosophies and what shapes trainers' expectations about how to deliver training. Students are also influenced by culture mediated through family expectations and contact with peers (Li, 2012).

Western cultures derive from ideas developed by Aristotle and Socrates, who focused on the individual. They prioritised critical reasoning and intellectual learning delivered through teaching, self-reflection and independent study along with humility and the ability to acknowledge mistakes. Eastern education is underpinned by Confucianism and its emphasis on moral cultivation. In Eastern traditions, what is important is to teach values and virtues that underpin harmony in human relations. These include self-restraint and good relationships through introspection and self-understanding. You and Rud suggest that 'by doing so, it helps to accommodate competing interests, needs, and values among people' (You and Rud, 2024: 100).

Brion reminds us that knowledge is contextual and that when educators are blind to cultural barriers, this can reduce the effectiveness of their training. She found that sensitivity to the cultural backgrounds of students 'would contribute to better academic, social, and emotional outcomes for all educators and students, regardless of race, ethnicity, gender, religion, sexual orientation, language, abilities, and cultural backgrounds'. In order to avoid a cultural mismatch Brion recommended that educators use a cultural lens in their planning, implementation and follow-up (Brion, 2021: 40–41). Conversely, it has been found that less culturally sensitive training is likely to reduce the student's capacity to apply new knowledge to their work. Caffarella and Daffron suggest that in order to provide quality training, educators need to develop culturally sensitive training materials (Caffarella and Daffron, 2013; Closson, 2013; Sarkar-Barney, 2004; Silver, 2000; Yang et al., 2009).

Learning is affected by cultural perceptions of time; cultural rituals associated with training (for example the value placed on certification and ceremony); students' perceptions of power differences, and the level of formality between student and trainer; whether the training included students from collectivist (Eastern) or individualistic (Western) cultures; and how comfortable students were in giving constructive feedback to the trainers. There was evidence that more sensitive attunement to cultural expectations improves learning transfer in professional learning (Brion, 2021: 41–43).

Students from cultures that value individualism are more likely to prefer 'active experimentation and abstract conceptualisation and reflective observation'. Holtbrügge and Mohr suggest that, 'If individuals from different cultural backgrounds have different learning style preferences, a one-size-fits-all model might be unlikely to help students achieve the required learning outcomes (Holtbrügge and Mohr, 2010: 633). Holtbrügge and Mohr recommend discussion about preferred learning styles with students to create a learning environment built on cooperation between students from different cultures. This can create an enriching learning experience (Holtbrügge and Mohr, 2010: 634).

Designing effective training that is culturally appropriate can be helped by:

- Trainers being curious about the cultural norms that may shape their students' learning.
- Trainers beginning by discussing the appropriateness of their approach to course delivery with the students.
- Trainers holding early discussions with the students about diverse practices.
- Trainers recognising that a trainer who relies solely on their own experiences when selecting material may be biased or less in tune with a diverse group of students.

Student diversity can be enriching. Tanaka studied experiences of communication between Japanese and international students. Participants highlighted the 'value of international perspectives, noting that these interactions enriched their understanding and boosted their confidence'. This was in spite of initial language barriers (Tanaka, 2025).

In conclusion, different cultural traditions need to be taken into account when offering training across cultural divides. Brion recommends that trainers provide pre-course preparation for students that takes account of culture when considering the context of the training, course content and materials (Brion, 2021: 43).

Ingredients that facilitate positive adult learning experiences

a) Learning from students

One of the main features of effective training is the quality of the relationship between trainers and students. Titsworth (2001) found a positive correlation between student learning and the trainer's level of engagement with the group. Students pick this up from verbal and non-verbal cues such as eye contact, smiling, the use of humour and tone of voice, and the trainer's friendliness and approachability (Titsworth, 2001). All these increased student engagement and learning long term. Additionally, effective trainers summarised the format for their presentation, used personalised examples and highlighted the key aspects. Sierens suggested that lesson structure may also improve self-regulated learning by students (Sierens et al., 2010).

O'Hair and colleagues concluded that good learning outcomes required both effective teaching *and* good listening skills by students. Better learning outcomes were also more likely when trainers engaged students by framing their input in the form of questions and answers and used examples that supported their application in the real world (O'Hair et al., 1988). Research by Thweatt and McCroskey found that students learned less well in response to trainers who did not hold their learning needs in mind. Students were less engaged when trainers arrived late, were unprepared, failed to keep to the syllabus or cancelled classes at short notice. This was confirmed by Marsh and Hattie whose research in a university setting found that trainers' expertise in their field did not in itself guarantee effective learning (Marsh and Hattie, 2002).

b) What does theory say about how students learn?

This section looks at how students learn, referring to Foulkes' approach with psychiatrists (Foulkes, 1964: 249–253), Prest's reflecting team supervision used by systemic therapists (Prest et al., 1990) and the Greek model of supervision, where the student group has no supervisor (Tsegos, 1995: 121). The section also touches on Stacey (2003) and power issues, and the concepts of 'reflection on action' and 'reflection in action'. Finally, the section combines these approaches to underpin the group analytic model described in this chapter.

In supervision, Foulkes encouraged students to think from three different positions—conductor, presenter and observer. Being able to give and receive feedback provided a series of mirrors on the work. The effect of each therapist's unique personality on their therapy groups became easier for each to see. Others were able to help them recognise when they had been pulled out of role in a countertransference enactment. Foulkes was able to recognise and formulate an understanding of what was happening when the supervision group was diverting their attention from their task. He was also focused on what was happening in the presenting therapist that was having an adverse effect on their behaviour in their therapy group (Foulkes, 1964: 251).

Systemic approaches like group analysis recognise the importance of the impact of social environment on us as individuals, shaping behaviour in a way that may be out of conscious awareness. 'In order to articulate implicit competencies and theories, any therapist needs to be seen from the outside. Here introspection is not enough, as implicit theories are embedded in what he does, rather than what he thinks about or reflects on' (Bertrando and Gilli, 2010: 21).

Bertrando and Gilli describe a way of reaching unconscious assumptions through observing behaviour rather than thoughts and feelings. In systemic supervision, the supervisor acts as a catalyst, encouraging peers to develop and present hypotheses about hidden assumptions in response to the behaviour they have observed. The presenting supervisee is the expert. Fellow peers are colleagues, who offer differing lenses through which the presenting supervisee can view their work. Change is the enlargement of perspective to include observation about the way things appear from the outside. This 'reflecting team process' involves two groups, who observe each other and offer feedback (Prest et al., 1990). This is the approach used with trainee supervisors on the IGA supervision training course to learn through observation and feedback. Parallel process is also much easier to recognise in the observer position, An account of a client who is raging will create a very different ambience in the group being observed compared with an account from someone who is mourning.

Scanlon applied two terms from Schon's theory of learning to supervision practice. Reflection-on-action happens when a case is presented from memory where conscious concerns are articulated. Reflection-in- action is when the group think about their experience in the here and now (Scanlon, 2000: 228). One of the aims of group supervision training is to foster this skill.

In Tsegos' Greek model, peers analyse the group material given by the therapist, sharing thoughts about the main themes along with feelings and fantasies. These are then processed by making links between the supervision group's reflections and the patient group material. When the group is blocked, they 'close the circle' to analyse the process in the here and now of the group (Tsegos 1995: 123). The Greek model has a structure that consists of three stages. They are the presentation, the analysis and the synthesis. After the presentation, the analysis phase identifies themes, and the group offer their feelings and associations. During the synthesis phase, the group make connections between the material from the therapy group and from the supervision group. They also make comments and suggestions (Tsegos, 1995: 122–123). These approaches are combined in the IGA supervision training and used in the reflecting team sessions (Smith and Gallop, 2023: 202–214).

c) The issue of power in supervision training courses

The issue of power is explored here because its impact has a significant effect on learning. Stacey describes learning as a process that involves the repeating of patterns of communication in the context of power relations. It is by this means that learning changes the identity of the people involved. Attention to where the power lies in training and how this may affect learning is always important. For Stacey, learning—the process of digesting information—cannot take place without the incorporation of power into this dynamic. This aspect will be further discussed in the section below that focuses on effective training. In addition to this, Stacey is highlighting the less considered impact of power inherent within the learning process (Stacey, 2003: 8). An observer watching a seminar may notice that some voices, and particularly that of the subject expert, carry more authority than others; and that some contribute more confidently than others.

Adults on training courses will come with their own, often considerable, expertise. When we learn something new, we risk of being seen as incompetent in the eyes of others, particularly those perceived to hold more expertise. This can create anxiety and can be deeply shaming. Trainers need to 'understand how people respond to the potential for shame' when facilitating the learning process because it closes down learning (Stacey, 2003: 9). Research into effective supervisors suggests that one of the key qualities they possess is that they are willing to be humble (Watkins, 2014). This capacity to be able to recognise their limits and to acknowledge that, in some areas, others may have more expertise and experience applies to trainers too. The capacity to do this in a humble way can help trainees to feel more willing to take risks in their seminars with their peers as they think together about their work.

Casemore stresses the importance of training for supervisors being far more collegial than in the approach adopted for the training of therapists (Casemore, 2018: 16–24). This is to reflect the seniority of the people joining the course. Participants in senior positions within their organisation can be fearful about being exposed and shamed when sharing their clinical work. Training courses that hold this in mind allow time to reflect on issues of power and authority in order to help participants reflect on how they use them within their own relationships. One opportunity for thinking about this during the IGA supervision training is when students are assessed.

Burck and Daniel suggest that supervisors may find it difficult to own the position of power they enjoy. They find it uncomfortable to be in a role where their words can be given special significance (Burck and Daniel, 2019: 158). When trainers show that they adapt to constructive feedback, they give course participants an experience of their own agency. When they model this, the course participants are more likely to model this in their own supervisory practice. It is easier for supervisees to acknowledge their difficulties in the work and think about their blind spots when their trainers, peers and their supervisors do the same.

d) Research into the training of supervisors

Most research is based on courses developed to offer dyadic supervision. Loganbill and Hardy highlight the importance of trainees offering supervision during training alongside their theory and skills development (Loganbill and Hardy, 1983: 15–21). Barrow and Domingo offered evidence that having a supervisor who had received supervision training enhanced supervisees' experience of supervision (Barrow and Domingo, 1997). Trained supervisors are more able to relinquish some control and allow their supervisees to be more active participants in the process. Research into group supervision of psychodynamic therapy for clinical psychology trainees found that, while there was some anxiety about exposing mistakes, overall it provided containment and a space for thinking and sharing experience. This increased confidence in interventions with clients (Hirschfeld et al., 2012). Henderson notes that there are many supervision training courses across the UK. (These are also largely courses in dyadic supervision). Henderson also notes that little has been written in this area, but it was evident that observed practice and feedback is viewed as essential to developing supervisory skills (Henderson, 2018).

Group analytic supervision training

The role of the supervisor is complex, and that of the supervisor of groups even more so. At its core, group analytic supervision training is the reworking of skills developed for working as therapists, adapting them to be appropriate for providing group supervision. For Foulkes, learning about group analysis was achieved through dialogue in groups, and this is central to learning that helps participants integrate their learning into their practice. The key to learning and change is effective communication. The skilful trainer is able to facilitate the student group communication as it moves from reflection on learning to applying it in practice appropriately in each part of the course.

What is important is to encourage diverse voices to create a rich tapestry of experience. The IGA supervision training is designed to maximise communication between students and trainers, space for conversations between students, discussion about the theory, and about practice and about how theory links with practice. The next sections bring a cultural lens to the course components.

a) The application process

Following the group model, the IGA supervision course starts with a group interview where potential course participants hold a conversation related to supervision training. The group interview is a good way to select supervisors who are comfortable with being in a group, able to listen to others respectfully, and who contribute in a collegial way while being able to draw on their own authority appropriately. Indication is given at interview that applicants are valued as experienced practitioners working in senior positions and that this itself provides much of the rich learning over and above the formal content of the course material.

After the group interview, applicants are interviewed individually to look in more detail at their readiness for the training. Bailey provides guidelines for readiness, including having built up enough of their own supervisory experience; having the capacity to offer an honest self-appraisal of their current motivation, ideally in discussion with their own supervisor; having sufficient training and qualification in the modality in which they will be supervising; and being comfortable with using their own autonomy (Bailey, 2009: 48–49).

b) The theoretical learning module

Theory is taught through reading and presentations from seminar leaders and students, along with skills development exercises appropriate to the topic. It covers group analytic concepts relating to group supervision, including the matrix, communication, translation, mirroring, resonance, polarisation, location, transpersonal processes and anti-group behaviour. Seminars focus on group analytic concepts as they apply to the provision of supervision in the group. The course covers dynamic administration (the boundaries and framework of supervision), supervisory relationships, unconscious processes, transference, countertransference and parallel process as they arise in group supervision. The course also revisits group dynamics and how difference contributes to the richness of the process. Students from individualistic cultures may find the reading component easier, although there may also be time pressure making this a challenge. People who are used to being taught may find the seminar input the most helpful while those from cultures that welcome discussion are more likely to thrive in any debate.

Power is invested in the course staff who select what they consider to be the most appropriate and up-to-date reading material for students. This is often an unnoticed power—for example, the decision to choose between two theoretical approaches, or to include both. An example of this would be using the model of the anti-group to understand difficult supervision group dynamics (Nitsun, 1996). Nitsun suggested that when groups are not carefully selected, the death instinct can give rise to fear and hostility, leading to anti-group behaviour. He then goes on to look at how this can be managed in order to use its creative potential. Another way of understanding challenging group dynamics would be to consider the influence of power in a group. Dalal talks about power as the generator of difference, and he sees the creation of insider and outsider dynamics as often underlying difficult dynamics in groups. In this approach, addressing power dynamics can help in working with tensions in groups (Dalal, 1998).

c) Reflecting team supervision

Reflecting team supervision fosters skills development through linking skills with practice. The reflecting team supervision blends Prest's concept of the reflecting team supervision model (where one group observes the other from behind a screen) with the concept of 'scenic understanding' developed by Albert Lorenzer (Lorenzer, 1974: 283). One member of the group holds the boundaries (as is the case for the training of students in Athens) (Tsegos, 1995: 122) while the therapist presents a 'snapshot' from their work that stirred strong feelings in them. This snapshot includes briefly describing the scene and naming the feelings evoked in them. The supervision group associate with this, observed by the reflecting team who then change places and give feedback. Following on from this, the two groups join together to process the experience. In order to make this a safe enough space, this part of the course is not assessed. Two supervision groups are formed on the first day of the course and the groups stay together for the duration of the course. A fuller description of this process can be found in Smith and Gallop (2023: 202–214). The essential ingredient here is 'teamwork', something that sits more comfortably with people from cultures that value collaborative approaches to learning.

d) Integration of theory with practice

Some past students have found this the most challenging part of the course. The session meets in two small groups to focus on linking the theory they have been learning with their own supervisory practice through small group discussion. The task is to think about how theoretical formulations can help as a lens for elucidating both the supervision group process and the patient work. This is a less lively and more reflective process involving the capacity to think at an intellectual level as well as being about feelings and relationships.

e) The supervision of supervision module

The IGA training is a national course and some participants have also come from Europe. The IGA London supervision training is provided in five weekend blocks. The supervision of supervision arrangements[1] takes account of this by meeting face-to-face at each block, and then weekly between blocks using Zoom. The groups begin at the first block with a face-to-face meeting. The meetings at each block are important for establishing and maintaining the supervisory group alliance. Post-pandemic, much experience has now been gained in working this way. However, when disruption takes place, this can arouse attachment issues which may need to be contained by the group. Geographical distance, especially for countries where internet access is less reliable, may come into the spotlight if poor connections intrude on the supervisor space.

The task of the supervision of supervision groups is to support the trainee supervisors with their role. First, many trainee supervisors might need help with forming their supervision group and negotiating the dynamic administration. Second, the supervisor of supervision will support the trainee supervisors in thinking through any boundary or other dynamic administration in the context where the supervision group is taking place. Third, the supervision of supervision provides the space for each of the trainee supervisors to reflect on the work that the therapists who are in their supervision group are bringing. There can be much rich learning from observing others in addition to receiving feedback about their own work. The supervisor of supervision is expected to give feedback on progress and to write a report on the work of each student towards the end of the course. The students are also asked to give feedback on their experience of their supervisor. This can help in modelling learning about how to work with students in training for future supervisors who go on to train students.

f) The median group

The median group conductors have traditionally been the course directors. This provides an opportunity for them to get to know each cohort. They hold the boundaries and encourage communication, thinking and reflection, intervening to reduce confusion and help make sense of the group process when needed.

The two median groups per block provide students with a space to develop their capacity to think and communicate within the larger group. Course members can also bring their experiences from other parts of the course, to reflect on conscious and unconscious processes and their experience of the boundaries, and the dynamic administration of the course itself. They may also explore power, difference, rivalry, leadership and followership, mirroring, and creative and destructive phenomena, as they operate within the median group. It offers the opportunity to give and receive feedback from colleagues, and this can help with identifying their valency for taking up roles or positions in a group. This learning can be useful when reflecting on their supervisory role. Course participants come from a wide range of cultural, geographical and organisational backgrounds, with differing professional languages that contain within them the power relationships pertaining to their specific professional group. This is the place where these dynamics can be explored in more depth.

The larger size of group helps to make it a different experience from that of being in group analysis. The purpose of the median group is not to offer therapy, although it allows some limited opportunity for touching on personal issues, such as trauma and bereavement. This 'in between' space has parallels with the tension in supervision groups. The supervisor has to navigate between maintaining a focus on clinical work and responding sympathetically when personal crises such as illness, bereavement or work difficulties affect the therapists. The supervisor is responsible for finding a way to talk about what is going on for someone without turning it into therapy.

The median group can be used to check how far presuppositions have affected group communication. It also provides an opportunity for giving and receiving affirmation and support, another key ingredient of well-functioning supervision groups. Along with the student meeting at each block, the median group acts as a container for the course, providing a space to talk about things which have not been fully aired elsewhere.

g) Student meeting

Students meet with the course directors at each block to bring up any concerns. The students set the agenda, and the staff will follow up on queries where they are unable to give immediate answers. The meeting is brief, no more than 10–15 minutes. It ensures that there is a space for two-way communication. This can avoid student issues going unnoticed or getting enacted unconsciously.

h) The spaces in between

One of the benefits of block supervision training, as referred to here, is the use of the spaces in between. The provision of food at lunchtime and biscuits with coffee and tea in other breaks between each aspect of the course allows some free time in an otherwise intensive programme of learning together. The coffee breaks and the lunch breaks provide a space where therapists from different backgrounds and different parts of the country meet together less formally. This can add to the richness of the experience.

Conclusion

The IGA supervision training draws on Foulkes' approach to group supervision, where the therapist gains perspective through a series of lenses and not just from one person in the position of expert. It offers a model for providing effective supervision in a group, which values the expertise of the group and not just that of the supervisor. Students learn through actively engaging in conversations in each of the course components and in developing their supervisory skills through offering a supervision group with weekly supervised practice. While the demands of the course can be challenging and anxiety provoking, it provides a diversity of learning from an experienced staff team and course participants also benefit enormously from being with each other and learning together.

Group analysis and group analytic supervision are founded on the belief that culture is fundamental in shaping each of us and it is a place where difference is seen as having value. Although not always a comfortable experience, the course welcomes diverse experiences and perspectives from diverse cultures. We live in a multicultural society. Effective trainers show curiosity, cultural sensitivity and the capacity to support and engage students, alongside their interest and expertise in the field.

Note

1 The supervisors in training bring their supervisory work to the course. They have their own supervision for this in a group, facilitated by a supervisor who is a senior practitioner.

References

Bailey C (2009) *Recruitment and Access*. Karnac Books.

Barrow M and Domingo R (1997) The Effectiveness of Training Clinical Supervisors in Conducting the Supervisory Conference. *The Clinical Supervisor*, 16: 57–78.

Bertrando P and Gilli G (2010) *Mirrors and Reflections: Theories of Change and the Practice of Systemic Supervision*. Routledge.

Brion C (2021) Culture Impacts Learning—And Not Just for Students. *The Learning Professional*, 42: 40–43.

Burck C and Daniel G (2019) *Mirrors and Reflections: Processes of Systemic Supervision*. Routledge.

Caffarella RS and Daffron SR (2013) *Planning Programs for Adult Learners: A Practical Guide*. Wiley.

Casemore R (2018) It Is All in the Relationship: Exploring the Differences Between Supervision Training and Counselling Training. In: Henderson P (ed.), *Supervisor Training: Issues and Approaches*. Routledge, pp. 15–25.

Closson RB (2013) Racial and Cultural Factors and Learning Transfer. *New Directions for Adult and Continuing Education*, 137: 61–69.

Dalal F (1998) *Taking the Group Seriously: Towards a Post-Foulkesian Group Analytic Theory*. Jessica Kingsley.

Foulkes SH (1948) *Introduction to Group-Analytic Psychotherapy*. Heinemann.

Foulkes SH (1964) *Therapeutic Group Analysis*. George Allen and Unwin.

Foulkes SH (1990) *Selected Papers of SH Foulkes: Psychoanalysis and Group Analysis*. Karnac Books.

Hattie J and Marsh HW (1996) The Relationship between Research and Teaching: A Meta-Analysis. *Review of Educational Research*, 66 (4): 507–542.

Henderson P (2018) *Supervisor Training: Issues and Approaches*. Routledge.

Hirschfeld R, McDonald P and Williams D (2012) Practice Based Learning: The Impact of Psychodynamic Supervision Groups on the Development of Psychodynamic Clinical Skills. *Clinical Psychology Forum*, 1 (240): 27–31.

Holtbrügge D and Mohr A (2010) Cultural Determinants of Learning Style Preferences. *Academy of Management Learning and Education*, 9: 622–637.

Li J (2012) *Cultural Foundations of Learning: East and West*. Cambridge University Press.

Loganbill C and Hardy E (1983) Developing Training Programs for Clinical Supervisors. *The Clinical Supervisor*, 1 (3): 15–21.

Lorenzer A (1974) *Die Wahrheit der Psychoanalytischen Erkennthis: Ein Historisch-Materialistischer Entwurf*. Suhrkamp.

Marsh HW and Hattie J (2002) The Relation between Research Productivity and Teaching Effectiveness. *The Journal of Higher Education*, 73 (5): 603–641.

Nitsun M (1996) *The Concept of the Anti-Group*. Routledge.

O'Hair M, O'Hair D and Wooden SL (1988) Enhancement of Listening Skills as a Prerequisite to Improved Study Skills. *International Listening Association*, 2 (1): 113–120.

Prest LA, Darden EC and Keller JF (1990) 'The Fly on the Wall': Reflecting Team Supervision. *Journal of Marital and Family Therapy*, 16 (3): 265–273.

Sarkar-Barney S (2004) *The Role of National Culture in Enhancing Training Effectiveness: A Framework*. Emerald Group Publishing.

Scanlon C (2000) The Place of Clinical Supervision in the Training of Group-Analytic Psychotherapists: Towards a Group-Dynamic Model for Professional Education? *Group Analysis*, 33 (2): 193–207.

Schön DA (1987) *Educating the Reflective Practitioner: Toward a New Design for Teaching and Learning in the Professions.* Jossey-Bass.

Sierens E, Vansteenkiste M, Goossens L, et al. (2010) The Synergistic Relationship of Perceived Autonomy Support and Structure in the Prediction of Self-Regulated Learning. *British Journal of Educational Psychology*, 79: 57–68.

Silver D (2000) Songs and Storytelling: Bringing Health Messages to Life in Uganda. *Education for Health*, 14: 51–60.

Smith M and Gallop M (2023) *Group Analytic Supervision.* Routledge.

Stacey R (2003) Learning as an Activity of Interdependent People. *The Learning Organization*, 10 (6).

Tanaka H (2025) *Speaking Across Cultures: Understanding Communication Styles in International Education.* (Graduation thesis, under review). Tokyo University.

Thweatt KS and McCroskey JC (1998) The impact of teacher immediacy and misbehaviors on teacher credibility. *Communication Education*, 47 (4): 348–358.

Titsworth BS (2001) The Effects of Teacher Immediacy, Use of Organizational Lecture Cues, and Students' Notetaking on Cognitive Learning. *Communication Education*, 50 (4): 283–297.

Tsegos Y (1995) A Greek Model of Supervision: The Matrix as Supervisor—A Version of Peer Supervision Developed at IGA (Athens). In Sharpe M (ed.), *The Third Eye: Supervision of Analytic Groups.* Routledge.

Watkins CE (2014) The Supervisory Alliance: A Half Century of Theory, Practice, and Research in Critical Perspective. *American Journal of Psychotherapy*, 68: 19–55.

Yang B, Wang Y and Drewry AW (2009) Does it Matter Where to Conduct Training? Accounting for Cultural Factors. *Human Resource Management Review*, 19 (4): 324–333.

You Z and Rud AG (2024) The Philosophy of Chinese Moral Cultivation: Justification and Educational Implications. *Beijing International Review of Education*, 6: 86–103.

Chapter 10

The Supervision Group as a Liminal Space

Navigating Rites of Passage using the Clinical Hexagon

Maddy Loat

> ... All the world's a stage,
> And all the men and women merely players;
> They have their exits and their entrances,
> And one man in his time plays many parts...
>
> (Shakespeare, *As You Like It*, 1599)

This chapter was originally written as a qualifying paper for the Institute of Group Analysis (IGA) Diploma in Supervision: Using the Group as the Medium of Supervision.

Introduction

Drawing on Winnicott's concept of the transitional object (Winnicott, 1953), and its application to the supervision group (Schneider and Berman, 1991), I propose the supervision group can be regarded as a 'liminal space' that forms a portal between the multiple realms requiring attention. In many ways the work of therapy holds up a mirror to the life cycle and, in this chapter, I demonstrate how reconceptualising the supervision group as a liminal space supports successful navigation of the necessary 'rites of passage'.

With the aid of clinical vignettes, and using the group analytic model of the clinical hexagon (Smith and Plant, 2012), I will focus on how themes relating to developmental stages, including trauma and loss, were mirrored across the matrix and how this led to a new understanding of the supervision group space. To conclude, I propose the supervision group can be understood as a liminal space, a threshold between, where new ways of thinking and being can begin to emerge. This concept has helped me to understand more fully the unique potential the supervision group can offer in its application to therapeutic work.

Defining group supervision: key concepts

Contemporary psychoanalytic and group analytic psychotherapy are both built on the foundations of object relations theory. Supervision of both

DOI: 10.4324/9781032719085-13

approaches share common ground, yet there are key differences. In dyadic supervision, attention is focused on the dynamic between the patient being presented and the therapist (the transference), as well as what is being evoked in the therapist (the countertransference). The countertransference includes split-off parts of the patient's internal world, as well as the therapist's own lived experiences and what may be evoked in them by the therapeutic material. Alongside this, there is an additional layer involving the dynamic between supervisor and supervisee, which frequently mirrors aspects of the therapeutic transference.

The multiple layers involved in dyadic supervision illustrate how inherently complex supervisory work is. In group supervision this increases exponentially with the additional people and experiences involved. Supervision groups can often feel like being inside a giant kaleidoscope, the multiple positions and perspectives akin to a constantly shifting pattern of infinite possibilities. The sheer volume of information can feel like sensory overload, creating a significant challenge as to where to focus attention. The following theoretical models and concepts are helpful in this regard, functioning rather like navigational tools that sufficiently orient the supervisor so they can effectively support the group members and the therapeutic work.

The clinical hexagon

Smith and Plant (2012) introduced the group analytic model of supervision called the clinical hexagon to help make sense of the multi-layered material inherent in supervision groups. This draws on the work of Ekstein and Wallerstein and their model of the clinical rhombus (Ekstein and Wallerstein, 1958). Whereas the clinical rhombus has four corners—the patient, the therapist, the supervisor and the organisation; the clinical hexagon has six corners through the addition of two more dimensions: dynamic administration and the supervision group dynamics/process. In contrast to Ekstein and Wallerstein, Smith and Plant apply their model to group supervision rather than dyadic supervision.

The six facets of the clinical hexagon interact with and have an effect on each other (Smith and Gallop 2024). These facets consist of (1) the patient or group being presented; (2) the therapist who is presenting; (3) the supervisor's self and countertransference; (4) the organisational context; (5) dynamic administration; and (6) the supervision group process (which may parallel the therapy).

A group analytic model of supervision uses the supervision group as a medium for reflection on therapists' work. The clinical hexagon provides a framework for the supervisor to assist group members in maintaining a reflective stance under pressure. The model of the clinical hexagon builds on group analytic practice in the tradition of S.H. Foulkes. It provides the supervisor with a map to assist them to notice what is in the foreground of the group's attention and what may be missed because it has been in the background and unnoticed. Each corner of the clinical hexagon will have an impact on the content and shape of the supervision group discussion.

(Smith and Gallop, 2024: 95)

The clinical hexagon provides a compass for the supervisor and the supervision group to help keep their bearings, as they think about their reflections on a case. When supervisors notice that their supervision group have been going round in circles, or they have been travelling down one path to the exclusion of others, without seeming to get anywhere helpful, it offers alternative routes.

(Smith, 2016: 3)

Parallel process, resonance and mirroring

Searles introduced the concept of parallel process to describe how the supervisor's emotions reflect aspects of the therapy relationship (Searles, 1955). This was developed by Ekstein and Wallerstein, who proposed it is a two-way process, and by Caligor who detailed how emotions and attitudes are transmitted from the therapy relationship to the supervisory relationship and vice versa (Ekstein and Wallerstein, 1958; Caligor, 1984). Parallel process is closely connected to the group analytic concepts of resonance (Foulkes, 1990) and mirroring (Foulkes and Anthony, 1990). Foulkes described resonance as an instinctive and intuitive process. It is an interpersonal response when the inner world or emotional state of one person is in tune with that of another. Mirroring is similar to parallel process in that it also describes a projective process but differs in its focus. In contrast to parallel process, mirroring is instead concerned with what happens when one person in a group observes behaviour in another that either resonates for them or reflects a part of themselves they do not wish to accept. With regard to the latter, Zinkin developed this further by introducing the concept of malignant mirroring where each person appears to the other as that which they unconsciously project and are in denial of (Zinkin, 1983).

Bringing our focus back to the supervision group, the concept of location of disturbance (Foulkes, 1964) is useful in considering how these processes and experiences manifest between and within each individual member as well as in the group as a whole and in the wider matrix that the group sits within.

Location of disturbance

Foulkes proposed that the group itself forms a matrix inside which all other relationships develop.

This view holds it axiomatic that everything happening in a group involves the group as a whole as well as each individual member. In what precise way it involves any of them, or even which aspects of each are actually mobilized, is a matter of paramount interest. An unending variety of configurations, including the conductor in his particular position, can be observed. To this category of concepts belongs for instance the idea of a location of a disturbance in a therapeutic group.

(Foulkes, 1964: 49)

Although Foulkes is talking about the therapeutic group here, what he proposes can also be applied to the supervision group.

Transitional objects and transitional space

Winnicott (1953) introduced the term transitional object to describe an object created and discovered by the infant for comfort, employed to support the developmental necessity of separating from their primary caregiver (Winnicott, 1953). This 'serves as a bridge between that which is comfortably familiar and whatever is disturbingly unfamiliar' (Greenacre, 1969: 145). Schneider and Berman were the first to employ Winnicott's concept of a transitional object to the supervision group. In their study of supervision groups for student interns on psychiatric placements they concluded that, similar to a transitional object, the supervision group allowed for 'the exploration and expression of feelings relating to the conflictual bind, enabling the intern to cope with the dual roles of university student and agency professional' (Schneider and Berman, 1991: 65).

I agree with Schneider and Berman but suggest their ideas can be further developed by considering Winnicott's concept of shared transitional space (Winnicott, 1975). In my opinion, this concept has been seriously overlooked when considering the work of the supervision group. Winnicott believed that between the inner world and the outer world, there is an intermediate area, which he referred to as transitional space. Winnicott says, 'The intermediate area to which I am referring is the area that is allowed to the infant between primary creativity and objective perception based on reality-testing' (Winnicott, 1975: 8). This area lies between phantasy and reality and allows for the child's imagination and creativity to flourish. This space is not only a physical space, but also a psychological and emotional one and it provides the child with the freedom to play, to explore and to start to develop a sense of self. Winnicott emphasised the importance of transitional space in play and in psychotherapy (Winnicott, 1971).

I would argue that transitional space is also important to consider when thinking about clinical supervision and the supervision group. However, for the supervision group to work optimally it needs to function as a space in transition as well as a transitional space. This is where the notion of liminality and the concept of liminal space are key. Although a healthy supervision group undoubtably needs to play and to be given the necessary space for the integration of imagination and reality to coincide, it also requires being prepared to exist in a state between. To fully participate in group supervision requires a capacity to be in this in-between place, on the threshold between. This necessitates an ability to remain open in one's disorientation of being and not-knowing, to allow for the potential of change and metamorphosis to occur.

Liminality and liminal space

The word liminality comes from the Latin *limen*, which means 'threshold'. In anthropology, liminality was developed as a concept to explain the sense of ambiguity and disorientation arising from the middle stage of a rite of passage, where one is no longer their pre-ritual self but not yet their complete self after undergoing some sort of a metamorphosis (van Gennep, 1960 (1909); Turner, 1969). The contemporary artist James Marshall, who has devoted many years to creating what he refers to as liminal objects, states:

> If subliminal means that which is below the threshold of ordinary consciousness and perception, liminal is the point of emergence, the threshold itself, the turning point between one realm and another. The liminal state is characterised by ambiguity, openness and indeterminacy. Liminality is a period of transition, during which usual boundaries of thought, self-understanding and behaviour shift, opening the way to something new.
>
> (Marshall, 2006)

Chairs as transitional objects in liminal space

The function of chairs within liminal space is an important aspect to consider. Chairs hold a key role in therapy, as well as in the supervision group. In the supervision group they tend to be placed in a circle, symbolising the communal and collaborative nature of the group. Dalal argues that supervision needs to be 'constituted by reciprocity and mutuality', knowledge being emergent and co-created (Dalal, 2023: 79). In response, Bacha suggests close attention needs to be paid to the inherent power inequality in supervision to avoid abuses of power (Bacha, 2023). Historically, sitting has been associated with power. In many languages, the verb 'to sit' is employed to refer to positions of power, e.g., sitting president, chairman, etc.

The conceptual artist, Joseph Kosuth, in one of his best-known works, *One and Three Chairs*, presented his visual expression of Plato's Theory of Forms

(Kosuth, 1965). The piece consists of a wooden chair, a photograph of the chair, and a dictionary definition of the word 'chair'. According to Plato's theory (from the fourth century BCE), non-material abstract Forms (or ideas) are the most fundamental kind of reality, as opposed to the physical world (Plato, 1975).

I propose that chairs, in both symbolic and physical form within the liminal space of the supervision group, and within the wider matrix, offer valuable information that can help us better understand the unconscious processes that are central to the work of supervision. In my opinion chairs can be understood as transitional objects in liminal space, providing opportunities to sit in the in-between spaces as well as the means to move from one realm or stage to another. This is illustrated in the clinical material below where chairs are a recurring motif within the liminal space of the supervision group.

Group composition and organisational context

For the purpose of confidentiality all names and identifying characteristics of people and places have been changed.

The supervision group under discussion was part of a well-established third-sector organisation based in a large UK city offering low-cost, affordable therapy to adults living or working in the local area. At the time of writing, I had been working there for several years as a self-employed clinical supervisor, conducting supervision groups for trainee and qualified psychotherapists offering weekly individual psychodynamic psychotherapy for up to 60 sessions. Placements were for a maximum of five years, meaning trainees had the option of staying for a designated period beyond their psychotherapy training. The supervision group was slow-open (meaning when one group member left a new group member joined). There was a maximum of three members in the group at any one time. I had been running this particular supervision group for eight years.

At the time of writing, the membership consisted of one man and one woman with another woman due to join. Ali had been in the group for three years having completed his training the previous year. Dita, who was in her final year of completing a second psychotherapy training course, had been in the group for one year. The new member, Maya, had recently completed an entry level psychotherapy course and was joining to gain more clinical experience with a view to undertaking further training. We met in a designated room within the organisation for two hours every fortnight. During each supervision, all members, who worked with a maximum caseload of three patients each, would present their clinical work. The time was divided equally, and the group rotated every session, so each member had opportunity to present first, second and last. There was designated space at the start of each supervision for group members to bring back reflections from previous supervision as well as general issues needing to be discussed.

Vignette 1: Who's been sitting in my chair?

At the beginning of the group, I reminded Ali and Dita that the new member, Maya, would be joining next time. There was a short silence before they shared mixed feelings. They agreed it would be good to have a full group again as they were missing this since the last member left. In contrast they had enjoyed having extra time and admitted feeling anxious about how the new person may change the group. Dita turned to Ali and said, 'Perhaps I'll move round and sit in your chair?', adding jokingly, 'It will be an upgrade!' Ali laughed and Dita then said playfully, 'Maybe you could move round to Maddy's chair?' He shook his head, exclaiming, 'No way ... I can't think that far ahead.' As they talked, I was thinking about a family preparing for the arrival of a younger sibling and I put this to them. This opened space for Ali and Dita to think more about their respective positions in the group, and both realised their ambivalent feelings about movement and change. This particularly resonated for Ali, who, for several weeks, had been trying to avoid thinking about how long he was going to stay on placement.

Maya joined the following session. I noted that Dita and Ali had chosen to sit in new chairs. Dita was now sitting in Ali's old chair and Ali was sitting in the chair next to me. Maya sat in the chair that Dita had been in the previous week. I welcomed Maya to the group and, mindful of the importance of attending to the necessary tasks of dynamic administration in this first session together, I suggested we start with introductions, before discussing and agreeing the frame. In this group I also made them aware I was due to be starting an advanced training in group supervision and that, with their permission, I would like to take material from the group to the training, adding that all identifying information would be anonymised to ensure confidentiality. All responded positively. Ali said, 'I like the fact you're doing this ... even supervisors continue training.' Maya and Dita echoed this. Knowing I ran other groups within the organisation, Dita added, 'I'm pleased you asked us; we're the special children!'

In this first session with the full group, I spent time attending to the dynamic administration, which involved discussing and agreeing the boundaries and the frame (Behr and Hearst, 2005). This is important to create a space with sufficient holding and containment for the group to feel safe enough to do its work (Winnicott, 1971). I purposely did this transparently and collaboratively to promote and build a shared sense of responsibility and ownership. I was also mindful of modelling what the group members needed to pay attention to in their initial therapeutic work with their own patients. Similarly, in my first supervision of supervision group within the training, my supervisor modelled something similar to us and I noticed how this made me feel the group was a 'safe enough' space for me to start to bring myself in.

When I took these two supervision groups to my preliminary supervision of supervision groups, it resonated with how we were all feeling about the training. Pleased to be there, feeling a bit like the 'chosen children', but also full of trepidation and anxiety preparing for this unknown journey, as well as the inevitability of 'sibling rivalries' (Parker, 2020). Similarly, in the median group there were strong themes relating to what it meant to be undertaking the training, stepping into the shoes of our elders. For me, this was complicated by the fact I had recently lost my long-standing supervisor, a well-known group analyst who had died suddenly four months prior to the start of my training. In many ways he symbolised an 'analytic father' to me and other group analysts of my generation. I found myself becoming upset in the first median group and needing to share this. This evoked similar experiences in the group, relating to life stage and loss, which felt supportive and containing. After the first weekend of training, I realised how the ambivalence that my group members had spoken about in context of their developmental trajectories was something I, too, was struggling with. I was reminded of Bion's assertion that the possibility of change inherent in emotional growth and development is inevitably linked to fears of catastrophe, that there can be no change without loss (Bion, 1966; 2014).

In my supervision of supervision group, we reflected on the symbolism of the chairs in my supervision group. This brought to my mind the fairy tale 'Goldilocks and the Three Bears' (Southgate, 1971). The story involves a little girl called 'Goldilocks' who enters the home of a family of three bears (mother, father and baby bear) who have gone for a walk in the woods. She tries the three different sizes of bowls, chairs and beds, each time finding the ones belonging to baby bear 'just right'. Bettelheim proposed that fairy tales serve as a means for a child to understand and integrate aspects of their maturing personality (Bettelheim, 1976). Through exposure to this type of fantasy narrative the child can formulate and think about their unconscious hopes and fears. Alongside this, the child is given a means of expressing and understanding the inner self via projection in that it gives hope of a more mature personality that has conquered the problems of the present.

Applying this to my supervision group, the chairs became a projection of the group members' unconscious hopes and fears in symbolising the natural progression from student to qualified therapist, as well as to potential supervisors in the future. This dynamic was also being mirrored outside the supervision group, in my own experiences and throughout the wider system. Within the organisation, just as patients would need to leave at the end of their therapy, therapists (the group members) would need to leave placement as they progressed. In addition, the organisation had been going through a tumultuous period, resulting in a number of changes—including new people sitting in leadership chairs. This had initially created a lack of containment in the service, and felt like a loss, especially for people like myself who had been working there for many years. These experiences, along with a desire to create space for new ventures, had set me thinking about leaving, but somehow it never seemed the right time. As my supervisory training progressed it became clear I was feeling an anxiety relating to abandonment, which I will say more about later. Suffice to say, at this point I was starting to become aware of the chair that I needed to vacate in the future, alongside the new chair I had taken up within the training.

Vignette 2: Unseated—Goldilocks enters the waiting room

Maya had now been in the supervision group for a couple of months, and the group was working well together. It was Dita's turn to present first, and she brought in two of her patients, Betty and Rita. They were both in their 20s, with similar backgrounds involving trauma and abuse. Dita described feeling highly anxious as she had become aware that Betty and Rita had started to develop a relationship in the waiting room. She described how she had walked into the waiting room after Betty's session to find Betty and Rita deep in conversation. Seeing Dita, they both laughed, and Betty proceeded to act out the role of being Rita's therapist. Dita said she felt humiliated and derailed. Maya commented how she was thinking about this in context of how we frequently confused Betty with Rita in the supervision group and wondered what this meant. Ali said it made him think about pairing and what they may be taking flight from. I wondered how this may connect with Dita's struggle to hold her authority as a therapist, something we had been exploring in recent months. Dita said it was helpful hearing these comments, and it was resonating with how she felt about nearing the end of her training. She then talked about her struggles with authority in the context of her early life experiences and leaving her home country to come to study and work in the UK.

Maya then talked about her experiences of being 'unseated' in her work with one of her patients, Shana, a single mother in her 40s, who was experiencing significant disempowerment in her life. In her countertransference, Maya said she often felt controlled by Shana. She gave an example of how, during the previous session, Shana had complained about the clock ticking to such an extent that she (Maya) ended up getting up from her chair to remove the battery from the clock. Ali said this made him think about trying to stop time so she would never have to leave therapy. I was aware there was a parallel process here and voiced this, commenting that I thought there was a strong theme relating to anxieties about attachment and loss.

In my supervision of supervision group, we discussed pairing as an attack on therapy, wanting to overthrow the therapist as a defence against loss. Someone picked up there was a parallel process, in that it reminded them of how Ali and Dita had previously wished to remain a pair in the supervision group, not wanting to let a third member in. Paradoxically it was Ali and Dita, as the more experienced therapists, who frequently appeared to be struggling more than

Maya. This made me think again about the theme of absent parents. I was struck by how, in the here and now, in my role as supervisor and in their role as therapists, we were all trying to be present and 'good enough' parents. With the help of my supervision of supervision group I was beginning to see how the unexpected and sudden death of my supervisor, so close to the start of the training, had created something of a blind spot for me in being able to connect to this theme.

Vignette 3: Empty chairs—location of disturbance

I was unable to attend the previous supervision group because I had an unexpected and serious family emergency. I contacted the group members as well as the organisation clinical lead and we agreed that the group would meet as a peer supervision group and that the clinical lead could be approached if there was anything urgent. I was aware that Dita and Maya had responded whereas Ali had not.

The following group both Dita and Maya said they were pleased to see me back, whereas Ali remained silent. I asked how their peer supervision group had been and again, Dita and Maya responded while Ali made no comment. I wondered what was happening but decided to keep quiet and see what emerged. It was Ali's turn to present. He started by asking if I had read through his application for accreditation as the deadline for submission had been the previous day. This immediately made me feel frustrated as there had been a repeating pattern of Ali sabotaging the accreditation process, similar to his wish to avoid thinking about leaving placement. I replied that I was surprised to hear this as he had not made me aware he was sending anything or that there was a deadline for submission. He shrugged which increased my frustration and I noticed I was now feeling irritated and angry. During this exchange Dita and Maya were looking confused and concerned and said that they had not heard him talk about this either. As time was pressing, I said this required further exploration, but we also needed to hear about his patients.

Ali presented Lisa, a forty-year-old woman who had a history of severe trauma including repeated childhood sexual abuse (CSA). In recent months she had disclosed to Ali that she had been physically abused by her male partner. After further exploration this had culminated in a safeguarding being raised with subsequent police and social services involvement. Ali discussed how he was continuing to struggle with Lisa's repeating pattern of engaging then disengaging with him and the work. He added that the session before the last supervision had been very challenging and he was left feeling anxious that Lisa might leave therapy. Dita said, 'Yes … and Maddy wasn't here.' Ali remained silent. I asked if he was angry with me. There was a sudden change in his affect. Now looking directly at me, he said clearly, 'Yes, I am. You're always here and then when I most need you, you're not.' This led to thinking more about the parallel process involving our experiences in the supervision group and what was happening in the transference between Ali and Lisa.

When I discussed this in my next supervision of supervision group, I shared the relief I felt in Ali finally expressing his anger towards me. The other members agreed this shift connected to the theme of absent parents. We also explored how this contrasted with my previous tendency to get drawn in to doing too much looking-after at times, especially during the various crises involving Lisa, who was also struggling with issues connected to absent parents. This theme of absent parents could also be seen in the wider matrix, evidenced by the lack of containment and holding in the organisation. This made me further reflect on the anger I felt towards the 'absent chairs' within the organisation, as well as the chair my supervisor had vacated. After his death, I learned he had been extremely unwell for a significant period of time, but he had not disclosed the full extent of this to me, or it seemed, to anyone else.

In the subsequent median group on the supervisory training, there were themes relating to power, authority and trauma. Recent unexpected changes to the timetable, alongside the end of the training approaching, had created some unsettled feelings in my cohort and me. During this group I began to realise I had been unable to get angry with the two course convenors just as Ali had been unable to get angry with me. The group wondered if, in context of my supervisor's sudden death, I was avoiding getting angry with them through fear of potentially 'killing them off'. It was clear that a powerful parallel process was again at work, and I left the training weekend feeling that something was beginning to shift. I continued to explore this in my supervision of supervision group, and gradually came to the conclusion it was time for me to leave the organisation. This time it felt life affirming rather than deadly. With the continued support of my supervision of supervision group, I eventually made the decision that I would hand in my notice and tell my supervision group.

Vignette 4: Moving chairs—rites of passage

At the beginning of the next supervision group, I announced my leaving and gave notice of when this would be. There was a brief silence before Dita exclaimed, 'I wasn't expecting that!' Maya echoed this and wondered where I was going. Ali, who had recently ended his therapeutic work, looked stunned and said 'Wow ... I guess this means I really have to decide when I'm leaving.' I agreed, but stressed the importance of him making this decision based on what was right for him, rather than being a reaction to my leaving. I added it felt time for me to leave after many years of working in the organisation, that it had been a difficult decision to make as I enjoyed working with them, but it was right for me.

Dita then jumped in, saying she did not want a new supervisor and when her patients came to the end of their therapy, she would be off. This made me think about my own struggles finding and working with a new supervisor after my supervisor had died, prompting me to say, 'No one is dying here, I understand it feels difficult but it may be helpful working with a new supervisor.' Maya said 'It's life, isn't it? There's always going to be change.' This theme continued as we proceeded to discuss the therapeutic work. Maya talked about her new patient, a man who was very ambivalent and had missed his second session. Meanwhile, Betty and Rita were making good progress, now no longer pairing in the waiting room as a result of Dita gradually feeling more able to step into her own authority as a therapist. Dita reported that Betty had recently become worried about her older brother and kept focusing on his needs rather than her own. I inwardly wondered whether there was a parallel process here, thinking Dita may be worried about Ali. I decided to keep quiet and wait to see what emerged.

When it was Ali's turn, he said he needed our help in thinking about whether to stay or leave. Although he had come to the end of working with his patients there was the opportunity to take on some shorter-term work if he wished to stay longer. Dita said, 'I think if I were you, I would leave, but perhaps that would be self-sabotaging?' Maya said she saw it differently: Ali had been on placement for over four years now and she wondered whether it was the opposite, not leaving potentially being a self-sabotage. Ali looked thoughtful and said 'Yes, it's confusing.' He returned to the theme of absent parents and said he now realised I'd become something like a good parent to him, and he also had supportive siblings here. This was a new experience for him, and he was now beginning to understand why it felt so difficult to leave. He added he thought Maya was correct, if he stayed, he would be self-sabotaging, by not being able to separate. He asked Dita if she was worried about him. Dita nodded and said she could see herself in him, that she was feeling a pull to leave now to avoid the feelings he had described but she knew she wasn't ready yet. Ali said, 'Yes, it's tough … I remember when Tomas left … I really wanted us to end at the same time but I'm glad I stayed. Just as I didn't need to worry about Tomas, you don't need to worry about me. I'm beginning to feel more ready now, well, as ready as I'll ever be.'

During this supervision group I felt a mixture of hope and sadness. It was a reminder that there can be no meaningful attachment without loss. In my supervision of supervision group, one of my peers wondered if, on an unconscious level, Ali may have been staying to look after me. In addition to being the 'oldest child/sibling' in the group constellation, he was also the only male in the group. Ali's valency to take up a paternal role made sense on multiple levels. I reflected on the recurring theme of absent parents, including the unexpected death of my older male supervisor just before the beginning of the training, and what this had evoked within me and my supervision group as well as how it had resonated within the wider matrix. After careful consideration in my supervision of supervision group and through further discussions with Ali, Dita and Maya, we agreed that Ali needed to end his placement and leave the supervision group before I left. In the context of the work we had been doing in the supervision group, it felt important these significant transitions were this way around. Ali's rite of passage in this particular liminal space was almost complete, as was mine.

Conclusion

Although I had worked as a clinical supervisor for many years, the training provided a new lens, as well as a good working compass. Both have put me in a much better position when considering where to focus and what needs attention when working as a clinical supervisor. The experience of training also led to a new way of conceptualising the supervision group.

In this chapter I have attempted to demonstrate how common themes in therapy relating to developmental stages involving attachment and loss were mirrored across the lifespan of the supervision group under discussion, as well as between the different aspects of the clinical hexagon and the wider matrix, including my own developmental trajectory. This coalesced in a clear parallel process which led to a new way of understanding the supervision group. Conceptualising the supervision group as a liminal space, and the chairs as transitional objects, helped me to deepen my understanding of supervisory work and to navigate a 'safe enough' 'rite of passage' for my supervisees, who, in turn, were able to apply this to their clinical work with their patients.

These themes were echoed in the last weekend of the training. In my supervision of supervision group we talked about a mixture of relief at having made it to the end but also sadness in needing to say goodbye. There were similar experiences in the other groups over the weekend and I recall an acute feeling of loss when I realised our reflecting team supervision had ended and there was another group in its place. In the last median group of the training I spoke about how I had been sitting in the same room the previous weekend, attending the memorial of my supervisor, a year since his death. Now a different stage, as I looked around the circle, I became aware we are all passing through these liminal spaces, and are changed by each other as we go. As we ended, I thought about who the chairs had held, and how they will continue to hold those of us who believe in the power of groups. When we leave, we take this and each other forward, as well as leaving something of ourselves behind.

Acknowledgements

I would like to express my gratitude to my supervisor, Peter Mark, and to my colleagues in my supervision of supervision group; the course convenors, Leonie Hilliard and Sara Perren; my personal tutor, Richard Curtis; and all involved in the 'Using the Group as the Medium of Supervision' Diploma Course. Thank you also to the members of my supervision group and to the organisation within which the group was held. The ideas in this chapter emerged as a result of the many shared interactions and discussions with all of the above.

References

Bacha CS (2023) Response to Farad Dalal's 'The Ethics of Supervision'. *Group Analysis*, 56 (1): 90–95.

Behr H and Hearst L (2005) *Group-Analytic Psychotherapy: A Meeting of Minds*. Whurr Publishers.

Bettelheim B (1976) *The Uses of Enchantment*. Random House.

Bion WR (1966; 2014) *Catastrophic Change*. Vol. 1. Karnac Books.

Caligor L (1984) Parallel and Reciprocal Processes in Psychoanalytic Supervision. In: Caligor L, Bromberg PM and Meltzer JD (eds), *Clinical Perspectives on the Supervision of Psychoanalysis and Psychotherapy*. Springer, pp. 1–28.

Dalal F (2023) The Ethics of Supervision: Reciprocity, Emergence and Prefiguration. *Group Analysis*, 56 (1): 62–80.

Ekstein R and Wallerstein RS (1958) *The Teaching and Learning of Psychotherapy*. Basic Books.

Foulkes SH (1964) *Therapeutic Group Analysis*. George Allen and Unwin.

Foulkes SH (1990) *Selected Papers of SH Foulkes: Psychoanalysis and Group Analysis*. Karnac Books.

Foulkes SH and Anthony EJ (1990) *Group Psychotherapy: The Psychoanalytic Approach*. Karnac Books.

Greenacre P (1969) The Fetish and the Transitional Object. *Psychoanalytic Study of the Child*, 24: 144–164.

Kosuth J (1965) *One of Three Chairs*. Artwork installation. New York City: Museum of Modern Art (MoMA).

Marshall J (2006) *Artist Statement*. Duane Reed Gallery. Available at: https://www.duanereedgallery.com/james-marshall (accessed 2025).

Parker V (2020) *A Group-Analytic Exploration of the Sibling Matrix: How Siblings Shape our Lives*. Routledge.

Plato (1975) *Plato's Phaedo*. Clarendon Press. (Original work written fourth century BCE.)

Schneider S and Berman M (1991) The Supervision Group as a Transitional Object. *Group Analysis*, 24 (1): 65–72.

Searles HF (1955) The Informational Value of the Supervisor's Emotional Experiences. *Psychiatry*, 18 (2): 135–146.

Smith M (2016) A Group Analytic Model of Supervision. (Unpublished).

Smith M and Gallop M (2024) *Group Analytic Supervision*. Routledge.

Smith M and Plant R (2012) Group Supervision: Moving in a New Range of Experience. *The Psychotherapist*, 50: 14–15.

Southgate V (1971) *Goldilocks and the Three Bears*. Penguin Random House.

Turner V (1969) *The Ritual Process: Structure and Anti-Structure*Aldine.

van Gennep A (1960; first published 1909) *The Rites of Passage*. University of Chicago Press.

Winnicott DW (1953) Transitional Objects and Transitional Phenomena. *International Journal of Psychoanalysis*, 34: 89–97.

Winnicott DW (1971) *Playing and Reality*. Penguin Books.

Winnicott DW (1975) *Through Paediatrics to Psychoanalysis: Collected Papers*. Routledge.

Zinkin L (1983) Malignant Mirroring. *Group Analysis*, 16 (2): 113–126.

Part 4

Professional Issues in Group Supervision

Chapter 11

Some Thoughts on Planned and Unplanned Endings

Margaret Gallop

Introduction

The nature of endings in group supervision can impact ongoing work and the outcomes of therapy. This chapter pays attention to the dynamic administration, structure and process of a satisfactory ending. Early experiences of loss among the group members and subsequent internalised expectations of unplanned endings may influence the lived experience of the supervision group endings. Endings impact on the legacy of the group in the minds of its members and could affect future ability to attach in professional relationships. The experience of a secure base and the opportunity to share important feelings within the work of the group can be internalised and support future supervisory relationships. The chapter pays attention to considerations for the group supervisor during transitions and endings.

In a therapy group, beginnings and endings, as well as members arriving and leaving, have a noticeable impact on the supervision group, more so when the supervisor leaves and another one comes in their place. Each of these events has an impact on the dynamic matrix and tests the important holding and containing structure of the supervision group. It may be important to bring them into the psychological awareness of the group. The changes may be thought of from a number of perspectives including the impact on the work, political impingements or its impact on relationships in the group, but the feelings around them are particularly important to acknowledge. The way the supervisor manages endings may also be absorbed as a model to be used in the therapy group that each member is conducting.

Theoretical perspectives

A group analytic approach

A group analytical perspective values the dialogue between group members in a supervision group, offering different professional, cultural and personal

DOI: 10.4324/9781032719085-15

perspectives. It considers the powerful influence of the particular family we were born into, how much we are 'steeped in its culture and language, which we consider to be natural' (Behr and Hearst, 2005: 261). Different reactions to the same complex material are represented by different members (Foulkes, 1964: 290). A well-functioning family seeks to have sufficient strength, cohesiveness and steadiness to weather arrivals and departures, and so will an established, well-functioning supervision group

Attachment perspectives: the supervision group as a secure base

John Bowlby's work on attachment theory introduced the concept of a secure base, a relationship from which the small child ventures out and to which they can return to recover themselves after experiences in the wider world. Within this relationship the child feels free to express their thoughts and feelings, including protest. This secure attachment has been used as a model for a therapeutic relationship (Wallin, 2007: 26).

Internal working models

Attachment theory suggests that what happens in these early years will contribute to the formation of an internal working model (IWM) of what is likely to happen in the wider world. If the child has had a responsive and attuned parent, they have the chance of developing secure patterns of attachment. If the parent or carer has been non-responsive or unpredictable and distressing, the child may have developed avoidant or ambivalent attachment (Wallin, 2007: 26). Where the parent or caregiver shows a still face the infant is likely to withdraw (Marrone, 1998: 205). These patterns can follow into adulthood and have an impact on adult behaviour in parenting and as adults in the workplace. Where the adult has the ability to trust and the colleagues and organisation are trustworthy then the supervisory process is supported. The process of supervision asks the therapist to be open about their work and continuously develop their self-awareness and reflect on their practice. The supervisor also continuously monitors their work and asks for feedback from their supervision group. Challenge is part of the supervisory process, and this is helped by building a culture of increased interactive understanding, words chosen with care and the building of trust. A supervision group can provide more responsive understanding and colleagues who can resonate with the material presented. The supervisor may then observe the process and understand more about the group dynamic mirroring the material being described. Where there is a less supportive organisation or group culture the therapist can feel exposed and less able to concentrate on client work and grow in professional development.

Starting a supervision group

The beginning of a group is a critical stage, where anxiety levels will be high, and members unsure what is about to happen. The supervision group is somewhere to bring self-doubt, confusion and dilemmas as well as sharing their clients' development. Members who have never been in a supervision group before may fear exposure after the privacy of individual supervision. This may temporarily override feelings of anticipation and excitement about the potential of the group to offer the support, multiple perspectives and learning for its members. This is where it is so important for the supervisor to focus their attention as the supervisor is the person responsible for dynamic administration, the management of both the internal and external boundaries of the group. Within negotiated boundaries, the group can become a source of professional belonging and acceptance, a place where new insights are available and creative options generated, a place of secure attachment in which important nurturing relationships are able to flourish.

Through the setting of the boundaries for the supervision group, the supervisor of groups models the way the therapist sets boundaries within their therapy group. This will include the way they will manage expectations about the way that endings and beginnings will be managed—for example, giving a notice period or advance notice of new people joining. This can then be referred to again when endings and new beginnings arise.

Growing a facilitating culture

A supervision group creates its own culture designed to support effective work with clients and groups. Members may be influenced by experience with previous supervision groups or individual supervision. What happens in the current group leaves a legacy that impacts on the next, carrying forward a culture like a yeast that can be grown again to make further bread. Good yeast can be passed from generation to generation. If it deteriorates it is important that it is discarded. The group supervisor pays attention to the early stages of the supervision group, which are formative and, like early life experiences, can set the trajectory for what is to follow. The supervisor may be internal or external to the organisation. They may take on an existing supervision group with its existing culture or set one up from scratch. In this chapter, I give examples of endings that challenge the supervision group's self-regulation and ability to sustain the work of the therapist.

Vignette A: An early leaving

Phil has been asked to start a new supervision group in a voluntary agency working with young people, where Jim, an older man, is part of the group of therapists in training. It is soon found that Jim finds it hard to keep clients, has limited training and may be unready for the work. Previous jobs have not been with people. The organisation arranges that Jim will leave, with the suggestion of other possible ways forward with young people or further training. But Jim has been a valued member of the group for his personal qualities. The supervision group members respond to his moving on by providing a home-made cake made by one of the members. The group, who did not know the full story, were able to honour Jim as a person and say goodbye with some sadness.

Discussion

Although the member had not been able to fulfil their task for the organisation, they were able to leave with dignity; and, although anxiety was raised, the way the group dealt with the leaving enabled the group to continue without a sense of diminution.

Jim who had some secure attachment from his upbringing was able to take the feedback and leave with dignity to decide whether or not he wanted to pursue further counselling training. The cake could be viewed as a gesture of ambivalence, but Zinkin commends ending rituals as they have always been part of human society (Zinkin, 1994: 83).

If the aim of therapy is to create the sense of a secure base in the client (Holmes, 1997: 167), encouraging secure attachment in the supervision group can further this. In his address 'Too Early, Too Late: Endings in Psychotherapy', Holmes explores further the match between the therapist and the client, how insecure, avoidant or ambivalent attachment may play out in the ending stages. If anxiety is lowered in the supervision group, these anxious responses may be less likely to interfere with steady thinking about what the client or group needs. 'A good ending is possible once a secure base has been established' (Holmes, 2001: 139).

Further reflection

Jim was a member of a supervision group within a voluntary organisation. How a volunteer leaves has an impact on the group. There is scope for insecurely attached volunteers to experience anxiety about how the organisation will deal with the rest of the volunteers in their supervision group. A member leaving a supervision group can be experienced as a loss. The closeness that has been developed could lead the departure to feel like a diminution of the group or an erosion of its value. The departure may resonate in different ways with each group member who may have experienced early or recent loss. It may echo with work that is ongoing in the group and so be amplified. All these outcomes provide possible amplification of feelings in the supervision group. Here, Jim had felt respected within his supervision group and had good support outside of his role as volunteer, giving him the resilience needed to move on with confidence. If Jim had defended himself by being dismissive about the group this could have been experienced as an attack, diminishing the group's understanding of itself.

Here the organisation has a role as a container for the supervision group. If surrounding circumstances were not containing and supportive, the group may be impacted. For example, if the organisation is under threat, there may be a fear of overall disintegration, as if a ship is taking on water. Once a boundary has been breached, fears can arise that others may follow. This may derive from members' previous unhelpful experiences in family or workplaces where similar things have happened and departures have not been handled well.

The group supervisor Phil decided to model containment and show that a departure is a survivable experience. He pointed out that when notice is given the counsellor or therapist can share their plans to leave and a last date can be agreed. The group can share in the sense that the member is going on to something good. That they are opening a good route that others may follow. In Jim's case, as someone with previous experience in accountancy, he had applied for and been accepted to train as a debt counsellor.

Vignette B: A healing experience

A therapist, Ahmed, joins a newly forming supervision group in a community setting staffed by trainees. He has previously had a bad experience in a supervision group in another part of the country where he felt his work was not valued, but he was unable to understand why. He had gone on to take part in a research project about destructive supervision. Ahmed takes a while to settle into the new supervision group, and noticeably ensures that his feedback to other members is given thoughtfully. It is a year before a review allows Ahmed to tell the supervisor about a previous demoralising experience of supervision and how healing he is finding the new group where he feels respected as a valued colleague. This allowed him to rework in his mind his experience of ending in his previous supervision group.

Discussion

The nature of the work of therapy means that workers can feel judged on their personal as well as professional qualities. Sharing counter transference reactions is potentially exposing because it reveals something about the individual. This means that care has to be taken in how comments are expressed. A supervisor is also a transference figure and because of this, their words are often given greater weight than those of their peers. They choose their words carefully or may wait for the group to give the necessary feedback. Other members of the group are peers and can be a little freer in what they say because the presenter may feel more able to choose whether or not to accept their contributions. In Ahmed's previous supervision group, his feedback was treated as less important than that of more senior colleagues in the group, leaving him feeling inferior.

Vignette C: A supervision group closes due to surrounding losses

Elizabeth provides supervision for a third sector organisation that arranges parenting groups for adults with adolescent family members. The staff are trained and experienced and are building up an expertise. The groups take place in a building within walking distance of the city centre, which also serves young people. The group has run for many years and is proud of its effectiveness, which has been monitored throughout. Now funding for the building has been withdrawn as well as financial support for the groups.

Elizabeth, the external supervisor, had heard the news of the closure of the service from the group members themselves, Franky, Benjamin and Charley. Other staff in the building had also been given notice of redundancy. There was shock and sadness and a concern for those young people whose parents were already in the group and for the bleak prospect for those on the growing waiting list. A group facilitator, Franky, blamed the charity for not planning ahead. Charley said it would be hard to face the parent groups with the news. Benjamin asked, 'What was the point of setting up imaginative projects?'
   The group feared this would lead to the end of the supervision group in its present form and that their work was not valued by the community. There was a growing sense of hopelessness. This was ironic because the counsellors had consciously cultivated a sense of hope in their groups. They had observed what a challenge this had been in a community that was disadvantaged in multiple ways.
   Elizabeth gave the supervision group time to express their feelings of disappointment, hopelessness and anger. This rekindled their determination to carry on to complete what had been promised to the current groups. During the last few sessions fixtures and fittings were moved out of the building, leaving the setting itself feeling like an uncomfortable place. Meanwhile the supervisees heard of a protest among those waiting to join the groups and that the waiting list had grown even longer. Although frustrated at not to be able to respond, they found it heartening to hear that their work had been valued.
   Elizabeth noticed some parallel process. The charity providing the groups was being deprived of the resources to carry on supporting the therapists and groups. This echoed many of the client families where the parents were endeavouring to muster the resources to bring up their adolescents. Elizabeth mentioned her perception of the parallel process in the supervision group and the members were able to discuss how this dynamic could have an impact on the members' work. By naming it, the dynamic had less power and it enabled the staff to think further about their thoughts and feelings and put these into words.

Individually they were able to approach the remaining sessions more helpfully. Franky was able to see that this blaming the organisation was a way of splitting off their anger and directing it onto the charity. Charley began to recognise her pattern of avoidant attachment with a tendency to withdraw that was part of a pattern of avoidance built from difficult experiences in childhood. Charley decided they could face the group and complete the sessions. Benjamin recognised echoes of his childhood deprivation. Identifying these feelings in themselves helped them to identify them in each group's members after they had broken the news and help them to talk about them. The therapists found an image of themselves holding together like a lift shaft in a building being demolished, often the last structure to go before the last remains of the building are bulldozed to the ground. This reinforced the view that their work was valued.

Discussion

With the opportunity to discuss their feelings, the group facilitators were able to weather the last few weeks of their groups. Differing attachment styles showed in their different responses. Although going separate ways, the group continued to meet informally for coffee to compare notes and support each other in new ventures. Having internalised the secure base of this supervision group as a good object, each found ways to continue their valuable work in the city, setting up groups elsewhere, pursuing further training and training others or by writing about it. There was a satisfaction in devising and sustaining ways of continuing the work in other settings.

Vignette D: Taking over a supervision group whose supervisor has left

Irene, an inexperienced supervisor, takes over a supervision group in a community counselling agency she is not familiar with. She is not informed about the circumstances of the previous supervisor leaving. The first group is difficult. The three members do not seem willing to accept a replacement. Irene finds that her encouragement to share their work is met with resistance. She decides to begin with a focus on the supervision group itself and encourages them to share their experience of their previous supervisor and acknowledge the loss they are feeling. Instead, the group present themselves as individuals with separate concerns and explain themselves via their different modalities and paths to the group. It seems that their relationship with the former supervisor had been providing containment of different views, which the transition was rekindling. They need to spend time getting to know Irene before they can feel safe enough, that their differences can be contained within their group. Irene accepts their anxiety that she may not be able to do this. At the second meeting the anxiety appears to have diminished, and they are able to share some of their work. Irene finds out later that the previous supervisor had left on maternity leave.

Comment

If a supervisor leaves to have a baby, strong feelings may be aroused. Cynthia Rogers wrote about her experience of having maternity leave from her analytic group, who reacted with strong transferential feelings of envy towards both the growing baby and the mother herself. Would the baby be taking away the mother's attention from them? Although at one level they were reassured that she was looking after herself and the baby by taking leave, there was resentment. How could she 'get on with her life' and leave them behind (Rogers, 1994: 55)? Would she be taking all the 'goodness, creativity and potency' of the group with her? (Rogers, 1994: 57). Maternity arouses strong transferential feelings that need to be acknowledged, to prevent acting out or being confused with case material. In this case, unexpressed feelings of loss and abandonment explained the lack of welcome Irene experienced.

Any change of supervisor may bring to the surface underlying tensions that had been quiescent. Are the members rivalrous? Would their competence be in question? Transitions heighten levels of anxiety and groups can fragment when the containment of familiar facilitator is lost. They may fear a loss of their accepted role and status. Will their work be understood and appreciated as much as by the previous person? They may feel a loss of visibility as a respected voice in the group. As the group member forms a supervisory alliance with a new supervisor, there will be some level of renegotiation of relationships within the group. In this case, the previous supervisor had given them a sense of belonging that had required her presence. In her absence they doubted their sense of value and effectiveness. They needed to share their backgrounds with the new supervisor, to test whether she would respect and accept them. After this test, it became possible for the group to reform with a new sense of safety and belonging.

Discussion

The response to change will be both individual and a shared group dynamic. If a therapist is at an early stage in their career, they may become partly dependent for their sense of effectiveness on being a member of this particular supervision group. The supervision group becomes a place where they are visible, accepted and respected. If they are older and nearer retirement the therapist may fear a loss of status in the group.

In her supervision of supervision group, Irene (the supervisor from Vignette D) wondered with the other group members whether a change of supervisor may benefit this particular group as they move away from their dependence for recognition upon a much-loved supervisor. She was helped to see that, as a new supervisor, she could bring different perspectives and, in doing so, she might be able to broaden their understanding of their own skills and value as therapists and reveal different defences and blind spots. She suggested that a change of facilitator can allow the group to explore issues that have been dormant (Rogers, 1994: 58).

Breaks in a member's presence

Breaks in attending a group may arise under a variety of circumstances. This section of the chapter explores breaks in attendance as a part of the dynamic administration that the supervisor will need to work with in the supervision group. Each event will raise its own unique considerations, each needing exploration within their supervisory work. The supervisor will need to balance competing needs, with the dynamic of the supervision group itself being weighed alongside the needs of the therapists to reflect on their work. The examples here include managing sickness absences, unexpected departures and retirement.

Ill health

When a group member takes a break, it may have a conscious and unconscious effect on the ongoing group. If someone is sick there may be a projection that they are being sick for the group, taking on the role for everyone. Their return may bring a sense of relief.

Unplanned departure

A sudden leaving can feel like negligence, rejection or abandonment.

Retirement

This could be the retirement of a therapist or the retirement of the group's supervisor. Every supervisor must at some point decide to stop. This may be because of ill health or incapacity, as well as outside factors, such as family issues or wanting to move on and explore the world in another way. Ill health leading to retirement raises important issues about disclosure or non-disclosure (Jacobs et al., 1995: 265). The decision to retire, particularly if it is forced by health issues, is a painful one. Giving up a profession that allows a sense of effectiveness, of contributing to the lives of others and of gaining insights and enrichments, can be painful. Others by contrast, may find the prospect of retirement liberating. The vignette below gives an example of the retirement of the group supervisor.

Vignette E: Decisions about endings and retirement

Pearl had run a supervision group for ten years. She felt it was going well, very much enjoyed her work and had a slow turnover of members. Having trained as a group analyst in her fifties she wished to continue as long as possible. But an unexpected diagnosis of a long-term illness, which would get gradually worse, could not be ignored. She wanted to do the best thing for her group, but also wanted to take her own feelings and the practicalities into consideration.

Initially, she hesitated to talk about her situation, anxious about response she might get. She had observed that sometimes friends encourage retirement without considering the full range of feelings this arouses. Among colleagues it could evoke peer group rivalry, both envy of those who retire and of those who continue to work. She decided to take her dilemma to her supervision of supervision group, consisting of experienced colleagues, facilitated by a younger supervisor, Bill. She put her hesitation aside and laid out her thinking. How could she make a professionally responsible decision? She assessed that in retiring she would be losing parts of her life at many levels. She would miss the reward of working closely with clients both individually and in groups and seeing them thrive. She would miss the status of being in a role where others listened to her views. This did not always happen in other situations. She would miss the rewarding as well as challenging relationships with her peers in the supervision group and their reciprocal support over many years. She would miss the social aspects of working. These last, she told herself, could in time be replaced. Retiring would mean multiple losses, which would require mourning and grieving. From her therapy she knew she had been brought up to think of the needs of others before herself. She did not want to repeat this unthinkingly.

However, would staying on with diminished health be the best professional decision for her groups? Would they pick up on her increasing frailty, which could affect what and how presentations were made? Or were her age and experience an advantage in a profession which took long steady learning. She knew that she was a transferential figure. Could she bear to renounce the wisdom they had imbued her with?

The group supervisor Bill thanked Pearl for bringing up this issue so openly. The group were shocked and sad to hear her diagnosis, and said they would miss her. They were proud to be her colleagues and remembered her past struggles as an ethnic minority woman in a largely white profession. The group discussed this at length, praising her work. Pearl was impatient about these compliments.

'I don't have any magical powers, just some experience.'

Jack, another older therapist, said 'I think someone quoted Prospero in relation to the retirement of therapists. When Prospero resigns his magical role in *The Tempest* he said, "Now my charms are all overthrown and what strength I have's mine own, which is most faint"' (Shakespeare, 1988/1611: line 1189).

Pearl referring to *The Tempest* too, replied 'My main contribution has been to be there, present in all weathers. There is nothing magical about that.'

Joan, another member, said, 'This is what I dread. It gets more difficult to stay well and get around.'

Jack, who had given the group notice that he is retiring soon, said 'They now think that *The Tempest* was written around the time Shakespeare retired and went back to his home town. That's what I'm going to do.' He paused, 'My father did that and said it was the best time of his life.'

Pearl, referring to her newly diagnosed long-term illness, said 'Now my family never had that choice', meaning that she felt her health condition would not allow her to retire to the rural area of the country she came from, but also she could not afford to stay where she was if she stopped working. She wondered how this was affecting her thinking.

Another member, Joan, said 'But if you want to keep going Pearl? You have so much to offer. The issue is whether to tell your groups you are ill or to keep it to yourself.'

'I had a supervisor who didn't tell us she was ill and she died suddenly,' said Jack. 'It was a terrible shock.'

Pearl remembered with a start that her mother had concealed a painful illness in order to keep her job.

Bill asked, 'What have you made of the discussion?'

Pearl thanked him. 'There is a lot to think about. How family experience is influencing me without my realising it. I may talk that through with someone. And I need information about the process of my illness, and when treatments might affect my thinking. How long will I be fit to practice, clear headed?'

Bill thanked Pearl and suggested that the group continue to support her in reviewing her situation.

Following this session, Pearl's colleague Jack brought his supervision group to a stop in the following year and left the group to fulfil his retirement plans.

Discussion

Bill reflected that this was a difficult subject for Pearl to bring and for the group to discuss openly and sensitively. 'The issue was pertinent to other members too. He could see that Pearl was full of strong conflicted feelings. He felt reassured that Pearl was trying to face the reality of her situation, planning to research the illness and treatment and seek support as well as continuing to bring the issue to group supervision. He pondered on how her cultural and family members' experience, the social unconscious, could be useful here (Zinkin, 1994).

Rogers points out the importance of staying in the real world when considering illness (Rogers, 2004). Anne Power has researched the area of therapists' retirement (Power, 2016) and suggests that the supervisees and patients have a conscious and unconscious understanding that the supervisor is unwell and may adjust their behaviour accordingly, being less challenging or robust in their demands. Unconscious reasons to continue may include a reminder of mortality (Power, 2016: 151), that retirement is a precursor of our eventual end. Power found that those with plans for their retirement found the transition easier.

Considerations around planning an ending for a supervision group

A functioning supervision group will at some stage either be brought to an end or passed over to another group supervisor. Facing reality and attending to practical issues is important. Some considerations are listed below.

- Keep communication going with any agency or organisation involved.
- Let the group know in good time.
- Allow time to talk about the ending and respect feelings of loss.
- Allow the opportunity for each member to express their responses including protest.
- Members may want to mention implications for their career and future plans.
- Make clear whether members can contact you again.
- Make sure the administrator knows, so room bookings match your plans.

How is the ending experienced?

Louis Zinkin in his journal article, 'All's Well that Ends Well. Or Is It?' (Zinkin, 1994), about the last stages of a therapeutic relationship suggests that it is very hard to know what has really happened. The ensuing unconscious and conscious continuation in the therapy client are hard to fathom and may contribute to personal development over time in an internalised dialogue (Zinkin, 1994: 16). Similarly, the supervision group may continue as an internal dialogue between the former members of a supervision group after the group has ended. Zinkin distinguished ending and stopping. Ending implies a completion, goals reached, whereas stopping does not. He suggests that, in managing the ending process, the analyst needs to stop interpreting, return gradually to reality and change to a different kind of conversation (Zinkin, 1994: 17). The supervisor of groups may also affect the type of conversation held at the end of a supervision group. Their contribution to the supervision group dynamics may be less interpretive with an increase in thinking about the realities involved in ending, as Zinkin suggests. The group's focus on their work may also include an element of review and consolidation. Perhaps when this is the case, a well-functioning supervision process, group or individual, continues on, like yeast carried inside each therapist to new situations.

Conclusion

If a supervision group is seen as a harbour where ships come in for a repair, replenishing resources and the restoration of the crew, the harbour walls need to be strong enough to withstand the outside ocean and the weather beating around the harbour. That may include occasional impact from badly piloted boats. It may be useful to learn of submerged rocks.

The setting may have complex dynamics from its location and population. The supervisor may not know everything about the underlying dynamics. Each arrival and departure in a supervision group has an effect on the supervision group members and requires attention and the opportunity to put feelings into words. The role of the supervisor in transitions and endings is critical and can model an approach for the therapists in their own work. Clarity and planning in the dynamic administration of the group can create a boundaried structure and setting. The care, respect and thoughtfulness become available, continually creating and also containing the group. This means that the group can accommodate some exposure and the risk of shame. It requires professionalism and generosity on the part of the members. In a well-functioning supervision group, a good enough experience of these fundamental qualities can be a platform supporting members when they leave the group, either because they are moving on to different work or to retirement.

References

Behr H and Hearst L (2005) *Group-Analytic Psychotherapy: A Meeting of Minds.* Whurr Publishers.

Foulkes SH (1964) *Therapeutic Group Analysis.* George Allen and Unwin.

Holmes J (1997) 'Too Early, Too Late': Endings in Psychotherapy—An Attachment Perspective, *British Journal of Psychotherapy*, 14 (2): 159–171.

Holmes J (2001) *The Search for the Secure Base: Attachment Theory and Psychotherapy.* Routledge.

Jacobs D, David P and Meyer D (1995) *The Supervisory Encounter: A Guide for Teachers of Psychodynamic Psychotherapy and Psychoanalysis.* Yale University Press.

Marrone M (1998) *Attachment and Interaction.* Jessica Kingsley Publishers.

Power A (2016) *Forced Endings in Psychotherapy and Psychoanalysis: Attachment and Loss in Retirement.* Routledge.

Rogers C (1994) The Group and the Group Analyst's Pregnancies. *Group Analysis*, 27 (1): 51–61.

Rogers C (2004) *Psychotherapy and Counselling: A Professional Business.* Whurr Publishers.

Shakespeare W (1988/1611) *William Shakespeare: The Complete Works: Compact Edition.* Oxford University Press. (Original work written 1611.)

Wallin DJ (2007) *Attachment in Psychotherapy.* Guilford Press.

Zinkin L (1994) All's Well that Ends Well. Or is it? *Group Analysis*, 27 (1): 15–24.

Chapter 12

Informing and Vitalising Group Supervision Practice

A Review of Research Evidence

Aisling McMahon

Introduction

Regular engagement in clinical supervision is a well-established and central aspect of training as a mental health professional, involving the mentorship and oversight of experienced professionals. Post-qualification attendance is also required for statutory or voluntary regulation for some professions in some countries, as part of clinical governance and maintenance of ongoing professional development (e.g., for counselling and psychotherapy in the UK and Ireland, and for psychology in Australia; see Hawkins and McMahon, 2020). Even when it is not a legal or professional requirement, having regular, good quality clinical supervision has been identified by practitioners as critical to maintaining resilience in frontline work, with high levels of engagement (McMahon and Errity, 2014).

Although clinical supervision has a central place and a long pedigree within the helping professions, practitioners traditionally took on a supervisory role by virtue of experience within their professional field, there being no acknowledgement of specific competencies needed for supervisory work. However, there has been a significant shift of perspective over the last 10 to 15 years, such that there is now international and interdisciplinary recognition of clinical supervision as a professional practice in its own right, requiring specific training and agreed standards of practice (Falender et al., 2014; Watkins and Wang, 2014). There has also been an exponential growth in the literature on clinical supervision, including an increasing range of books on supervision in different practice modalities (*Group Analytic Supervision* being an example of this; Smith and Gallop, 2023), as well as a surge in research publications (Watkins, 2011, 2020). All of this is of great value to inform best practice in supervision, but it is widely agreed that continued study is needed to understand the complexities of supervisory work within different modalities and contexts (Goodyear et al., 2016).

In this chapter, I first offer a broad overview of research on clinical supervision, followed by a more detailed review of research on group supervision, including studies that have compared individual and group supervision

DOI: 10.4324/9781032719085-16

formats, explored supervision group dynamics, and that have informed us regarding the group supervisor's role and competencies. In closing, I will offer some take-away points from the research to inform and vitalise group supervision practice.

An overview of clinical supervision research: What have we learned so far?

Research on clinical supervision can be broadly categorised into studies of experiences and impacts for clients/service users, supervisees and organisations, and investigations of specific aspects or modes of supervisory practice.

Researching the impact of a practitioner's supervision for their clients is challenging given that so many other factors influence client outcomes. As a result, there have been inconsistent findings to date, with some studies evidencing a strong impact (supervisors accounting for 16 per cent of the variance in client outcomes; Callahan et al., 2009; Wrape et al., 2015) and others finding no appreciable impact (accounting for less than 1 per cent of the variance; Rousmaniere et al., 2016; Whipple et al., 2020). A recent meta-analytic review concluded that the evidence to date is that clinical supervision has a small but significant contribution to client outcomes (4–6 per cent overall; Keum and Wang, 2021). However, most of these studies did not consider the nature of the clinical supervision, and some well-designed, longitudinal studies with differences in the regularity and focus of supervision offer a more nuanced picture. The findings of such studies suggest that more frequent supervision focused on developing particular skills is related to better client outcomes (see research review in Hawkins and McMahon, 2020). A good example of this is an Australian study, where clients of therapists who had weekly supervision focused on the therapeutic alliance did significantly better than clients of unsupervised therapists, with reduced symptoms of depression and less treatment dropout (6 per cent versus 31 per cent drop out; Bambling et al., 2006).

There is a stronger evidence base for the benefits of clinical supervision for supervisees. Practitioners from diverse disciplines and contexts report a range of benefits, including increased skills, knowledge, self-efficacy, development of professional identity and stronger client relationships (e.g., McAnally et al., 2022; McMahon and Hevey, 2017; Tan and Chou, 2018). In addition, a number of studies have reported greater professional competence in the recorded practice of those attending supervision following training, compared to those without supervision (e.g., Alfonsson et al., 2020; Rakovshik et al., 2016).

There is also good evidence of benefits for organisations and employers, as well as for their staff. Attending clinical supervision has been significantly related to greater job satisfaction (Carpenter et al., 2013; Dawson et al., 2013), improved emotional wellbeing and less burnout (Wallbank, 2013), and fewer sick days (Hyrkäs et al., 2001). However, again it is important to note that not all clinical supervision is equal, and supervisees have reported experiencing high levels of inadequate and harmful supervision (Cook and Ellis, 2021; Ellis et al., 2015). With this in mind, it is not surprising that stronger clinical supervision relationships that are experienced as more supportive or more effective have been related to higher work satisfaction, decreased work-related stress and lower levels of burnout (Livni et al., 2012; Poulin and Walter, 1992; Sterner, 2009).

Many other studies have focused on investigating important aspects of clinical supervision, including the supervisory relationship, power dynamics, feedback and evaluation, supervisor cultural competence and humility, and the application of supervision models to different practice contexts, to name a few (e.g., Crockett and Hays, 2015; Kovič and McMahon, 2023; McKibben et al., 2019; McMahon et al., 2022). Research into clinical supervision continues to develop in its scope and diversity, and this is invaluable for developing awareness and standards across supervisory contexts and modes.

A focus on some key areas of group supervision research

Many theoretical and clinical practice articles have been published regarding group supervision, offering guidance to understand and harness the potential of the group format (e.g., Berman and Berger, 2007; Kalai, 2007; Knott, 2016; Kutter, 1993; McMahon, 2014a; Moss, 2008; Rosenthal, 1999; Yerushalmi, 1999). Books and book chapters have also been written on group supervision, offering maps and models for practice (e.g., Beddoe and Davys, 2016: Chapter 7; Benson, 2025: Chapter 15; Hargaden, 2016; Hawkins and McMahon, 2020: Chapter 10; Page and Wosket, 2015: Chapter 9; Proctor, 2008; Sharpe, 1995; Smith and Gallop, 2023). However, research on group supervision has lagged behind the theoretical literature. In my own recent systematic narrative review of group analytic literature on supervision, I found that nearly all publications were theoretical and clinical descriptions of practice, there being only a few research studies (McMahon, 2023). A preponderance of small qualitative, exploratory case studies has also been highlighted in past reviews of group supervision research, and there have been calls for a broader range of methodologies to systematically explore and enhance our understanding in this area of practice (Francke and de Graaff, 2012; Holloway and Johnston, 1985; Mastoras and Andrews, 2011; Prieto, 1996).

It remains the case that small, exploratory interview studies of experiences in particular supervision groups are the most common type of research endeavour in this area, and these are an important contribution to building our knowledge from across different contexts. In addition to this work, the breadth of research approaches has developed over the years to include larger survey studies, detailed observational studies analysing recorded practice, longitudinal studies investigating impacts and experiences of supervision groups over time, as well as studies comparing group supervision with other types of supervision or the absence of supervision. Reviewing all the research to date is beyond the scope of this chapter but I will focus on some key studies in a few areas of research that I believe are useful for practitioners to be aware of—studies of differences between individual and group supervision, those exploring group supervision dynamics, and those that highlight important group supervisor competencies.

Individual versus group supervision

Group supervision has been described as the most frequently used modality during psychotherapy training in many countries (Boëthius et al., 2004), others describing it as a close second to individual supervision (Enyedy et al., 2003). Group supervision is also a popular mode of ongoing support and development for qualified practitioners (on its own or in combination with individual supervision, e.g., McMahon and Errity, 2014). Many clinical and theoretical publications have summarised the relative advantages and disadvantages of group supervision compared to individual supervision (e.g., Prasko et al., 2022; Proctor, 2008) but we also have some research studies comparing these modes in different contexts.

A few early studies compared the type of supervision attended in terms of impact on US trainee counsellors' development and skills. Lanning (1971) found no difference for trainees attending either individual or group supervision in their perceptions of their supervisory or counselling relationships, or in their clients' perceptions of their therapeutic relationships. Averitt (1988) also found no differences in empathic responding in the observed practice of trainees attending either individual or group supervision. Another study divided counselling trainees into three groups, one receiving large group supervision (8:1 trainee to supervisor ratio), one receiving small group supervision (4:1), and one having combined large group and individual supervision over a ten-week period. It was found that all supervision formats resulted in similar progress in counsellor effectiveness and development, as rated by the trainees, their supervisors, their clients and observers (Ray and Altekruse, 2000).

Other studies have focused on the experiences and impacts of qualified practitioners attending workplace clinical supervision with more mixed findings. In a survey of 260 UK community nurses, they perceived their supervision to be similarly effective whether they attended individual or group supervision, or a combination of the two (Edwards et al., 2005). However, a recent survey of nearly 1,000 Australian practitioners in violence and sexual assault services found that attendance at individual supervision (the most common modality), or a combination of individual and group supervision, were both associated with a lower intention to leave the service over the following year than attendance at group supervision alone (Cortis et al., 2021). In another longitudinal study, 42 staff in Australian addiction services, who volunteered to take part in the introduction and evaluation of workplace supervision, were allocated to either individual or group supervision (Livni et al., 2012). After six months, satisfaction with supervision and its perceived effectiveness were positively rated by both individual and group supervisees, although individual supervision achieved higher ratings. Also, highly rated individual supervision was significantly related to lower levels of burnout and higher levels of wellbeing and job satisfaction, while group supervision was not.

As can be seen, while equivalent benefits have been found for trainees attending either mode of supervision, for qualified practitioners there is more evidence in favour of individual supervision, or a combination of individual and group supervision, over group supervision alone. It has also typically been found that trainees prefer individual supervision. For instance, US social work students reported that group supervision provided socioemotional support and rich learning opportunities but that they felt less vulnerable in individual supervision, enabling them to more openly develop self-awareness and insight into their client relationships (Walter and Young, 1999). US student counsellors also preferred individual supervision, experiencing it as safer, deeper and more challenging, with feedback in group supervision being less personal, open and constructive, albeit offering valuable opportunities for vicarious learning and normalisation of concerns (Borders, 2012). Being more at ease in individual supervision was also reported by some qualified staff in a survey study of supervision in a UK healthcare setting, although other staff preferred group supervision, noting its contribution to staff cohesion and wider perspectives (Barriball et al., 2004). In another study, nurses in a Danish psychiatric hospital were interviewed regarding staff's limited participation in group supervision (Buus et al., 2010). Supervision with colleagues was described as 'uncomfortably exposing', the authors concluding that individual supervision might be more suitable in this work context. Research with Norwegian general hospital nurses also found that less than one-third of the participants attended group supervision regularly, but that those who did so experienced less workplace anxiety and an enhanced sense of control (Bégat et al., 2005).

Continued research is needed to investigate the relative benefits and challenges of individual and group supervision, extending into more diverse training and work contexts. Furthermore, the evidence of supervisees experiencing less safety, openness, depth, constructive feedback and challenge in group supervision points to the dynamic, relational complexities of this form of supervision, which has been an area of study in its own right.

The dynamic challenge of group supervision

Much of the research to date on group supervision dynamics has explored supervisee experiences, some studies also including supervisor experiences. Two survey studies with US psychology students identified helpful and hindering experiences in group supervision. Five categories of helpful events were identified: supervisor impact (e.g., open and validating style, competent and even-handed personality), specific instruction (e.g., the supervisor's expertise or use of in vivo techniques), self-understanding, support and safety, and peer impact (e.g., peer validation and constructive feedback) (Carter et al., 2009). Hindering events were categorised as between-member problems (e.g., competitiveness, criticism and non-participation), problems with supervisors (e.g., domineering style or inexperience), supervisee anxiety and other negative effects, logistical constraints (e.g., room size, time of day), and poor group time management/not enough time (Enyedy et al., 2003).

Another study explored experiences of learning, trust and competition in group supervision through interviews with US social work students. The students described times of feeling frustrated, angry, vulnerable and silenced, but that generally conflict and competition between students did not emerge openly: 'It never got nasty. I think most of those feelings were under the surface' (Bogo et al., 2004: 19). The students' experience was of a cautious, self-protective seeking of safety and trust, expecting the group supervisor to facilitate positive group dynamics (e.g., containing monopolising, encouraging open communication about group relations), and to model and promote group norms about risk-taking and feedback.

Similar experiences of vulnerability, limited spontaneity and unexpressed conflicts were reported in longitudinal mixed-methods studies of supervision groups with Swedish psychotherapy trainees, along with the expectation that the supervisor would 'shoulder responsibility' for emotional dynamics in the group (Ögren et al., 2002: 170). It was also found that the supervision groups that initially reported more opposition and conflict showed more flexible patterns of interaction at later stages, indicating the value of encouraging more independent expression of ideas early on to counteract typical efforts to be 'nice' and 'pleasing' (Boëthius et al., 2004). Across all supervision groups, the trainees became a little more satisfied with their groups over time, although supervisors perceived more positive progress than supervisees did. The researchers concluded that supervisors may underestimate how inhibiting group dynamics can be for supervisees and that they may need to 'sharpen their attention concerning the group climate' (Ögren et al., 2014: 664).

Interviews with Canadian social work students and their supervisors also indicated the need to build trust and safety in group supervision, external barriers to safety being found to include members' prior histories with each other and internal barriers, including non-reflective and risk-averse group members (Sussman et al., 2007). Again, some discrepancy between supervisors and supervisees was observed, the supervisors having expected that the supervisees would already have the skills to function as effective members of a learning group, and the supervisees having expected that the supervisors would do more to facilitate discussions of difficult dynamics.

In addition to ongoing investigations of supervision group members' experiences, there have been some recent, detailed studies of recorded practice, involving valuable analyses of group dynamics in action. An 18-month study of a peer supervision group of Chilean psychotherapists highlighted the ubiquity of regressive group dynamics and resistance to productive work (Yasky et al., 2019). The researchers' analyses identified the impact of complex workloads, parallels between supervision and therapy dynamics, and the individual and group minds' limited capacity to process raw emotional experience. They reported that these issues led to anxiety, dependent or passive attitudes, avoidance and intellectualisation. They also identified aspects of good workgroup functioning, including shared upholding of responsibilities such as group contracting and structuring of time, tolerance of confusion and uncertainty, and regular reflection on group dynamics that were impeding the work.

In another study, incidences of rupture and repair were analysed in seven recorded sessions of group supervision with US psychology trainees (Eubanks et al., 2021). Only minor ruptures were observed, it being found that when the trainees disagreed with each other or their supervisor, they often used a combination of subtle confrontation and withdrawal behaviours to resolve the issue. Confrontation behaviours included some pushing back, rejecting the other person's ideas or defending their own position, and withdrawal behaviours included laughter, which seemed to smooth over difficult moments, deferential behaviour and minimal responses. A notable finding was that tensions within the group were seldom named or explored, the supervisor typically resolving issues through providing a rationale, validating supervisee defensiveness or redirecting.

A discourse analysis of power dynamics in three recorded supervision group sessions in a UK child and adolescent psychotherapy clinic provided further insights (Lee and Thackeray, 2023). Productive, power-sharing supervisory discourses were observed to include empathic and cooperative expressions, cultivating room for individual ideas and group reflection. When discourses highlighted power differentials (e.g., involving interruptions or theory-based assertions), interpersonal conflicts and defensiveness were more likely to occur, restricting the flow and depth of group conversations. The researchers noted that this was more often observed in a predominantly male supervision group, with a predominantly female supervision group showing more attentive, empathic and responsive communication. As in Eubanks et al. (2021), it was observed that supervisors missed opportunities to initiate processes of repair or reflection at times of supervisee defensiveness or uncertainty.

Another recent study of recorded sessions analysed changes in group dynamics over a 14-session supervision group with Turkish counselling and guidance trainees, evidencing similar stages to those identified for therapy groups (Tümlü and Ceyhan, 2023). Initial dynamics were found to involve concerns about belonging and trust, with expressed feelings of incompetence, uncertainty and anxiety. A second stage involved more dissatisfaction, conflict, subgrouping, competition and resistance. A third 'working' stage evidenced a more dominant desire for development, closer and more trusting relationships, and more peer feedback and support. A final 'termination' stage was reported as involving self-evaluation, mixed feelings of comfort and sadness, and signs of independence as well as dependence on the supervisor, with some resistance and regression. In contrast to the previous two studies, these authors identified supervisor behaviours that had usefully contributed to the group navigating each stage of development, including contracting and clarifying goals, normalising conflict and resistance, self-disclosure, offering both support and challenge, and encouraging peer support.

Given the complex and often inhibitory dynamics evidenced across various studies on group supervision, further research is reviewed below where study findings offer direction regarding the group supervisor's role in facilitating good group functioning.

Competencies and skills needed for supervising groups

Research studies have identified various aspects that group supervisors need to attend to in facilitating effective group work, as well as some key group supervisor skills.

In setting up supervision groups, there is evidence indicating the value of carefully considering group size and composition. Gender differences were found in the discourse analysis study reviewed earlier, these researchers also observing that when there was a gender imbalance in supervision groups, those of the minority gender were more silent (Lee and Thackeray, 2023). Studies with Swedish psychotherapy trainees also found that having a gender balance had a positive impact on supervision group functioning, and that a group of less than four members negatively impacted trust and acceptance (Boëthius et al., 2006). Too much heterogeneity in these groups was also found to negatively affect security (Ögren et al., 2002). In another study with US counsellor trainees, supervision groups with differences in personal and professional backgrounds were valued in bringing multiple perspectives, but differences in experience level were perceived as detrimental, resulting in less experienced supervisees not always understanding feedback received and being less willing to share their own feedback or ask questions (Linton and Hedstrom, 2006).

Attention to contracting and clarifying boundaries in supervision groups has also been found to be important. A survey study with US supervisors and supervisees on ethical practice in group supervision reported strong agreement on the importance of establishing norms and structures for the work through contracting, attending to client confidentiality, privacy related to self-disclosures, discussion of evaluative procedures and management of multiple relationships (Smith et al., 2012). In support of this, a study of leaderless peer supervision groups found that groups that more competently attended to agreeing and reviewing goals and tasks were experienced by group members as more cohesive and worthwhile (Somerville et al., 2019).

Some relevant supervisor skills have also been identified through research. In interviews with experienced US group supervisors working across training and workplace settings, the group supervisor's self-awareness and ability to process multi-layered cognitive, emotional and behavioural factors in the group were emphasised, as well as the need to attend to potential parallel process dynamics (Atieno Okech and Rubel, 2009). Drawing from research on individual supervision, the importance of the group supervisor's multi-cultural orientation and sensitivity to privilege and oppression has also been highlighted (Peters and Luke, 2023; Watkins et al., 2022). While there has been a paucity of research in this area with supervision groups, one survey study which investigated US psychotherapy trainees' experiences of helpful and unhelpful multicultural events in their supervision groups offers some useful findings (Kaduvettoor et al., 2009). Mostly helpful events were identified, top ones being vicarious learning from peers, multicultural learning and multicultural conceptualisation in the group (e.g., becoming more aware of privileged identities). The most hindering events involved indirect discussion of cultural issues, cultural conflicts or disagreements with supervisors, and misapplication of multicultural theory (e.g., perpetuation of stereotypes). When hindering events occurred, the trainees expressed a wish for better integration of multicultural issues, and more supervisor involvement and interpersonal sensitivity.

Other research indicates that group supervisors need to explicitly attend to developing their relationship with their supervisees, as well as facilitating the development of peer relationships and group cohesion. A longitudinal study of Hong Kong counselling trainees' experiences of supervision groups found that both the quality of their peer relationships and of their alliance with their supervisor independently contributed to their satisfaction with supervision and their counselling self-efficacy (Chui et al., 2021). A similar finding was reported in Livni et al.'s (2012) Australian workplace study, where both supervisory alliance and group cohesion were equally predictive of perceived supervision effectiveness for group supervisees.

Some studies have offered more detailed insights into supervisees' experiences and management of difficulties in their relationships with their group supervisors. A survey study with Scandinavian psychology trainees found that they commonly coped with dissatisfaction with their group supervisor (e.g., due to perceived supervisor biases or inadequacies) through talking with the other supervisees outside of the supervision group, the researchers describing this as creating a 'common enemy' of the supervisor (Reichelt et al., 2009: 19). There were similar findings in interviews with Danish psychotherapy trainees about times of low alliance with their group supervisor (Hedegaard, 2020). Issues identified at these times were passivity or non-disclosure in the group, the supervisor being preoccupied with group dynamics, and either the supervisee or their supervisor being in an 'outgroup'. Again, separate discussions between supervisees outside of the group sometimes had an impact here, one supervisee perceiving her supervisor differently following feedback from the other supervisees: 'I looked at him with different eyes, or as if he is not just that listening, containing person, he is actually also kind of passive, reclining' (Hedegaard, 2020: 50). The supervisees also shared times of compensating for the group supervisor's perceived lack or lapses, the researchers noting ambivalent dependency-autonomy tensions in the supervisees' relationships with their supervisors.

These studies and the literature on group dynamics reviewed earlier evidence the need for group supervisors to have knowledge and skills in attending to group processes, openness and cohesion. However, a survey of 162 group supervisors of US psychology trainees found that while there was a high endorsement of the importance of working with group dynamics, there were wide variations in the time they gave to this (Riva and Erickson Cornish, 2008). One-fifth of the supervisors indicated that they never attend to group processes in their supervision groups, and another quarter reported doing so only occasionally. Those who did actively respond to group dynamics described doing so by facilitating process comments, relating supervision group process to clinical work, and encouraging supervisee self-awareness through discussing parallel process issues. It was notable that most of the supervisors (89 per cent) did not have specific training in group supervision, a surprising finding given the commonality of this mode of supervision. The need for focused training in this area was also identified in a survey study with Australian psychology trainees, whose supervisors provided both individual and group supervision (Grassby and Gonsalvez, 2022). In this study it was found that the trainees rated their supervisor's group supervision competencies (e.g., facilitating group engagement, ensuring safety for disclosure, and professional growth) significantly lower than all other supervisory competencies (e.g., openness, caring and support and therapeutic expertise and knowledge). Of course, this finding most likely reflects the added complexity of supervising groups, but again points to the importance of dedicated training for this work.

Key take-away points from research to inform best practice

Research regarding group supervision is still developing but some key take-away points from the evidence to date may be useful for group supervisors to be aware of in their ongoing practice:

- When setting up supervision groups, attention needs to be given to group composition and size given their impact on group functioning.
- As part of ethical practice, and to clarify expectations and roles in the initial stages of a supervision group, focused attention is needed on contracting for the group work, boundaries and relationships.

- Supervisees experience many benefits from group supervision but there is consistent evidence that they feel more vulnerable and inhibited in group supervision than in individual supervision so active attention to building safety and trust is critical.
- Encouraging supervisees to offer independent thinking and feedback, alongside typical efforts to please supervision group peers, can contribute to stronger flexibility over time.
- As a supervisor, it is important to attend to the development of stronger and more open relationships with each group member, as well as between group members, given that both vertical and horizontal relationships impact supervisees' satisfaction, self-efficacy and openness.
- Supervisor self-awareness and skill in attending to multiple group processes is required, including sensitive and regular attention to multicultural issues.
- A strong understanding of group dynamics is needed given that resistance and regression have been found to be common in supervision groups but are typically not directly expressed or reflected upon.
- Given the evidence that supervisees expect group supervisors to take responsibility for managing difficult group dynamics, and that supervisees may have less sophisticated group participation skills than supervisors expect, the onus is on the supervisor to lead and model more open communication, working to normalise, explore and productively work through challenging dynamics.
- Specific training in group supervision is important given the dynamic complexity of this mode of practice.

Concluding thoughts

I am greatly encouraged by the growth in the professional and research literature on clinical supervision in recent years, including a widening diversity of studies on group supervision. I have previously written about the impact of not having had clinical supervision early in my career when working with complex trauma in the Irish prison system, this work taking a higher toll than might otherwise have been the case (McMahon, 2014b). This experience was a driver for my own engagement in supervision research, and I have been keen to contribute to our knowledge of how best to support and foster resilient and capable practitioners. At this stage, much valuable research work has been done but more is needed to extend our awareness of the intricacies of group supervision practice in various training, workplace and disciplinary contexts. Such ongoing work will continue to strengthen group supervision's potential as a dynamic, vital and sustaining professional practice.

References

Alfonsson S, Lundgren T and Andersson G (2020) Clinical Supervision in Cognitive Behavior Therapy Improves Therapists' Competence: A Single-Case Experimental Pilot Study. *Cognitive Behaviour Therapy*, 49 (5): 425–438.

Atieno Okech JE and Rubel D (2009) The Experiences of Expert Group Work Supervisors: An Exploratory Study. *The Journal for Specialists in Group Work*, 34 (1): 68–89.

Averitt J (1988) *Individual Versus Group Supervision of Counselor Trainees*. Unpublished doctoral dissertation. University of Tennessee.

Bambling M, King R, Raue P, et al. (2006) Clinical Supervision: Its Influence on Client-Rated Working Alliance and Client Symptom Reduction in the Brief Treatment of Major Depression. *Psychotherapy Research*, 16 (3): 317–331.

Barriball L, While A and Münch U (2004) An Audit of Clinical Supervision in Primary Care. *British Journal of Community Nursing*, 9 (9): 389–397.

Beddoe L and Davys A (2016) *Challenges in Professional Supervision: Current Themes and Models for Practice*. Jessica Kingsley Publishers.

Bégat I, Ellefsen B and Severinsson E (2005) Nurses' Satisfaction with Their Work Environment and the Outcomes of Clinical Nursing Supervision on Nurses' Experiences of Well-Being—A Norwegian Study. *Journal of Nursing Management*, 13 (3): 221–230.

Benson J (2025) *Working More Creatively with Groups*. Taylor & Francis.

Berman A and Berger M (2007) Matrix and Reverie in Supervision Groups. *Group Analysis*, 40 (2): 236–250.

Boëthius SB, Ögren M-L, Sjøvold E, et al. (2004) Experiences of Group Culture and Patterns of Interaction in Psychotherapy Supervision Groups. *The Clinical Supervisor*, 23 (1): 101–120.

Boëthius SB, Sundin E and Ögren M-L (2006) Group Supervision from a Small Group Perspective. *Nordic Psychology*, 58 (1): 22–42.

Bogo M, Globerman J and Sussman T (2004) The Field Instructor as Group Worker: Managing Trust and Competition in Group Supervision. *Journal of Social Work Education*, 40 (1): 13–26.

Borders LD (2012) Dyadic, Triadic, and Group Models of Peer Supervision/Consultation: What are Their Components, and is There Evidence of Their Effectiveness? *Clinical Psychologist*, 16 (2): 59–71.

Buus N, Angel S, Traynor M, et al. (2010) Psychiatric Hospital Nursing Staff's Experiences of Participating in Group-Based Clinical Supervision: An Interview Study. *Issues in Mental Health Nursing*, 31 (10): 654–661.

Callahan JL, Almstrom CM, Swift JK, et al. (2009) Exploring the Contribution of Supervisors to Intervention Outcomes. *Training and Education in Professional Psychology*, 3 (2): 72–77.

Carpenter J, Webb CM and Bostock L (2013) The Surprisingly Weak Evidence Base for Supervision: Findings from a Systematic Review of Research in Child Welfare Practice (2000–2012). *Children and Youth Services Review*, 35 (11): 1843–1853.

Carter JW, Enyedy KC, Goodyear RK, et al. (2009) Concept Mapping of the Events Supervisees Find Helpful in Group Supervision. *Training and Education in Professional Psychology*, 3 (1): 1–9.

Chui H, Li X and Luk S (2021) Does Peer Relationship Matter? A Multilevel Investigation of the Effects of Peer and Supervisory Relationships on Group Supervision Outcomes. *Journal of Counseling Psychology*, 68 (4): 457–466.

Cook RM and Ellis MV (2021) Post-Degree Clinical Supervision for Licensure: Occurrence of Inadequate and Harmful Experiences Among Counselors. *The Clinical Supervisor*, 40 (2): 282–302.

Cortis N, Seymour K, Natalier K, et al. (2021) Which Models of Supervision Help Retain Staff? Findings from Australia's Domestic and Family Violence and Sexual Assault Workforces. *Australian Social Work*, 74 (1): 68–82.

Crockett S and Hays DG (2015) The Influence of Supervisor Multicultural Competence on the Supervisory Working Alliance, Supervisee Counseling Self-Efficacy, and Supervisee Satisfaction with Supervision: A Mediation Model. *Counselor Education and Supervision*, 54 (4): 258–273.

Dawson M, Phillips B and Leggat S (2013) Clinical Supervision for Allied Health Professionals. *Journal of Allied Health*, 42 (2): 10.

Edwards D, Cooper L, Burnard P, et al. (2005) Factors Influencing the Effectiveness of Clinical Supervision. *Journal of Psychiatric and Mental Health Nursing*, 12 (4): 405–414.

Ellis MV, Creaner M, Hutman H, et al. (2015) A Comparative Study of Clinical Supervision in the Republic of Ireland and the United States. *Journal of Counseling Psychology*, 62 (4): 621–631.

Enyedy KC, Arcinue F, Puri NN, et al. (2003) Hindering Phenomena in Group Supervision: Implications for Practice. *Professional Psychology: Research and Practice*, 34 (3): 312–317.

Eubanks CF, Warren JT and Muran JC (2021) Identifying Ruptures and Repairs in Alliance-Focused Training Group Supervision. *International Journal of Group Psychotherapy*, 71 (2): 275–309.

Falender CA, Shafranske EP and Ofek A (2014) Competent Clinical Supervision: Emerging Effective Practices. *Counselling Psychology Quarterly*, 27 (4): 393–408.

Francke AL and de Graaff FM (2012) The Effects of Group Supervision of Nurses: A Systematic Literature Review. *International Journal of Nursing Studies*, 49 (9): 1165–1179.

Goodyear RK, Borders LD, Chang CY, et al. (2016) Prioritizing Questions and Methods for an International and Interdisciplinary Supervision Research Agenda: Suggestions by Eight Scholars. *The Clinical Supervisor*, 35 (1): 117–154.

Grassby S and Gonsalvez C (2022) Group Supervision Is a Distinct Supervisor Competency: Empirical Evidence and a Brief Scale for Supervisory Practice. *Australian Psychologist*, 57 (6): 352–358.

Hargaden H (2016) *The Art of Relational Supervision: Clinical Implications of the Use of Self in Group Supervision*. Routledge.

Hawkins P and McMahon A (2020) *Supervision in the Helping Professions* (5th edition). McGraw-Hill Open University Press.

Hedegaard AE (2020) The Supervisory Alliance in Group Supervision. *British Journal of Psychotherapy*, 36 (1): 45–60.

Holloway EL and Johnston R (1985) Group Supervision: Widely Practiced but Poorly Understood. *Counselor Education and Supervision*, 24 (4): 332–340.

Hyrkäs K, Lehti K and Paunonen-Ilmonen M (2001) Cost-Benefit Analysis of Team Supervision: The Development of an Innovative Model and its Application as a Case Study in One Finnish University Hospital. *Journal of Nursing Management*, 9 (5): 259–268.

Kaduvettoor A, O'Shaughnessy T, Mori Y, et al. (2009) Helpful and Hindering Multicultural Events in Group Supervision: Climate and Multicultural Competence. *The Counseling Psychologist*, 37 (6): 786–820.

Kalai S (2007) Group Supervision of Individual Therapy. *Group Analysis*, 40 (2): 204–215.

Keum BT and Wang L (2021) Supervision and Psychotherapy Process and Outcome: A Meta-Analytic Review. *Translational Issues in Psychological Science*, 7 (1): 89–108.

Knott H (2016) Countertransference and Projective Identification Revisited and Applied to the Practice of Group Analytic Supervision. *International Journal of Group Psychotherapy*, 66 (3): 323–337.

Kovič D and McMahon A (2023) Building Trust: Supervisees' Experience of Power Dynamics in Transdisciplinary Workplace Supervision. *Journal of Social Work Practice*, 37 (4): 403–417.

Kutter P (1993) Direct and Indirect ('Reversed') Mirror Phenomena in Group Supervision. *Group Analysis*, 26 (2): 177–181.

Lanning WL (1971) A Study of the Relation Between Group and Individual Counseling Supervision and Three Relationship Measures. *Journal of Counseling Psychology*, 18 (5): 401–406.

Lee MC and Thackeray L (2023) Relational Processes and Power Dynamics in Psychoanalytic Group Supervision: A Discourse Analysis. *The Clinical Supervisor*, 42 (1): 123–144.

Linton JM and Hedstrom SM (2006) An Exploratory Qualitative Investigation of Group Processes in Group Supervision: Perceptions of Masters-Level Practicum Students. *The Journal for Specialists in Group Work*, 31 (1): 51–72.

Livni D, Crowe TP and Gonsalvez CJ (2012) Effects of Supervision Modality and Intensity on Alliance and Outcomes for the Supervisee. *Rehabilitation Psychology*, 57 (2): 178–186.

Mastoras SM and Andrews JJW (2011) The Supervisee Experience of Group Supervision: Implications for Research and Practice. *Training and Education in Professional Psychology*, 5 (2): 102–111.

McAnally K, Abrams L, Asmus MJ, et al. (2022) Coaching Supervision: A Study of Perceptions and Practices in the Americas. In: Seto L, Goldvarg D, and Eustice S (eds), *Coaching Supervision*. Routledge.

McKibben WB, Borders LD and Wahesh E (2019) Factors Influencing Supervisee Perceptions of Critical Feedback Validity. *Counselor Education and Supervision*, 58 (4): 242–256.

McMahon A (2014a) Being a Group Supervisor: Dynamics, Challenges and Rewards. *Inside Out*, 72: 21–32.

McMahon A (2014b) Four Guiding Principles for the Supervisory Relationship. *Reflective Practice*, 15 (3): 333–346.

McMahon A (2023) A Narrative Review of Group Analytic Literature on Clinical Supervision: Seeking Coherence and Correspondence. *Group Analysis*. Epub 27 February 2023. doi:10.1177/05333164231153927.

McMahon A and Errity D (2014) From New Vistas to Life Lines: Psychologists' Satisfaction with Supervision and Confidence in Supervising. *Clinical Psychology & Psychotherapy*, 21 (3): 264–275.

McMahon A and Hevey D (2017) 'It Has Taken Me a Long Time to Get to this Point of Quiet Confidence': What Contributes to Therapeutic Confidence for Clinical Psychologists? *Clinical Psychologist*, 21 (3): 195–205.

McMahon A, Jennings C and O'Brien G (2022) A Naturalistic, Observational Study of the Seven-Eyed Model of Supervision. *The Clinical Supervisor*, 41 (1): 47–69.

Moss E (2008) The Holding/Containment Function in Supervision Groups for Group Therapists. *International Journal of Group Psychotherapy*, 58 (2): 185–201.

Ögren M-L, Apelman A and Klawitter M (2002) The Group in Psychotherapy Supervision. *The Clinical Supervisor*, 20 (2): 147–175.

Ögren M-L, Boalt Boëthius S and Sundin E (2014) Challenges and Possibilities in Group Supervision. In: Watkins CE and Milne DL (eds), *The Wiley International Handbook of Clinical Supervision*. Wiley-Blackwell, pp. 648–669.

Page S and Wosket V (2015) *Supervising the Counsellor and Psychotherapist: A Cyclical Model* (3rd edition). Routledge.

Peters HC and Luke M (2023) Application of Anti-Oppression with Group Work. *The Journal for Specialists in Group Work*, 48 (2). Routledge, pp. 84–89.

Poulin JE and Walter CA (1992) Retention Plans and Job Satisfaction of Gerontological Social Workers. *Journal of Gerontological Social Work*, 19 (1): 99–114.

Prasko J, Abeltina M, Krone I, et al. (2022) Group Supervision in Cognitive Behavioral Therapy: Theoretical Frameworks and Praxis. *Activitas Nervosa Superior Rediviva*, 64(2–3):86–99.

Prieto LR (1996) Group Supervision: Still Widely Practiced but Poorly Understood. *Counselor Education & Supervision*, 35 (4): 295.

Proctor B (2008) *Group Supervision: A Guide to Creative Practice*. Sage.

Rakovshik SG, McManus F, Vazquez-Montes M, et al. (2016) Is Supervision Necessary? Examining the Effects of Internet-based CBT Training With and Without Supervision. *Journal of Consulting and Clinical Psychology*, 84 (3): 191–199.

Ray D and Altekruse M (2000) Effectiveness of Group Supervision Versus Combined Group and Individual Supervision. *Counselor Education and Supervision*, 40 (1): 19–30.

Reichelt S, Gullestad SE, Hansen BR, et al. (2009) Nondisclosure in Psychotherapy Group Supervision: The Supervisee Perspective. *Nordic Psychology*, 61 (4): 5–27.

Riva MT and Erickson Cornish JA (2008) Group Supervision Practices at Psychology Predoctoral Internship Programs: 15 Years Later. *Training and Education in Professional Psychology*, 2 (1): 18–25.

Rosenthal L (1999) Group Supervision of Groups: A Modern Analytic Perspective. *International Journal of Group Psychotherapy*, 49 (2): 197–213.

Rousmaniere TG, Swift JK, Babins-Wagner R, et al. (2016) Supervisor Variance in Psychotherapy Outcome in Routine Practice. *Psychotherapy Research*, 26 (2): 196–205.

Sharpe M (1995) *The Third Eye: Supervision of Analytic Groups*. Routledge.

Smith M and Gallop M (2023) *Group Analytic Supervision*. Routledge.

Smith RD, Riva MT and Erickson Cornish JA (2012) The Ethical Practice of Group Supervision: A National Survey. *Training and Education in Professional Psychology*, 6 (4): 238–248.

Somerville W, Marcus S and Chang DF (2019) Multicultural Competence-Focused Peer Supervision: A Multiple Case Study of Clinical and Counseling Psychology Trainees. *Journal of Multicultural Counseling and Development*, 47 (4): 274–294.

Sterner WR (2009) Influence of the Supervisory Working Alliance on Supervisee Work Satisfaction and Work-Related Stress. *Journal of Mental Health Counseling*, 31 (3): 249–263.

Sussman T, Bogo M and Globerman J (2007) Field Instructor Perceptions in Group Supervision: Re-Establishing Trust Through Managing Group Dynamics. *The Clinical Supervisor*, 26 (1–2): 61–80.

Tan SY and Chou CC (2018) Supervision Effects on Self-Efficacy, Competency, and Job Involvement of School Counsellors. *Journal of Psychologists and Counsellors in Schools*, 28 (1): 18–32.

Tümlü GÜ and Ceyhan E (2023) Clarifying the Stages of Group Supervision Through Action Research. *Anadolu University Journal of Education Faculty*, 7 (3): 479–499.

Wallbank S (2013) Maintaining Professional Resilience Through Group Restorative Supervision. *Community Practitioner*, 86 (8): 26–28.

Walter CA and Young TM (1999) Combining Individual and Group Supervision in Educating for the Social Work Profession. *The Clinical Supervisor*, 18 (2): 73–89.

Watkins CE (2011) Does Psychotherapy Supervision Contribute to Patient Outcomes? Considering Thirty Years of Research. *The Clinical Supervisor*, 30 (2): 235–256.

Watkins CE (2020) What Do Clinical Supervision Research Reviews Tell Us? Surveying the Last 25 Years. *Counselling and Psychotherapy Research*, 20 (2): 190–208.

Watkins CE, Hook JN, DeBlaere C, et al. (2022) Extending Multicultural Orientation to the Group Supervision of Psychotherapy: Practical Applications. *Practice Innovations*, 7 (3): 255–267.

Watkins CE and Wang CDC (2014) On the Education of Clinical Supervisors. In: Watkins CE and Milne DL (eds), *The Wiley International Handbook of Clinical Supervision*. Wiley-Blackwell, pp. 177–203.

Whipple J, Hoyt T, Rousmaniere T, et al. (2020) Supervisor Variance in Psychotherapy Outcome in Routine Practice: A Replication. *SAGE Open*, 10 (1). doi:10.1177/2158244019899047.

Wrape ER, Callahan JL, Ruggero CJ, et al. (2015) An Exploration of Faculty Supervisor Variables and Their Impact on Client Outcomes. *Training and Education in Professional Psychology*, 9 (1): 35–43.

Yasky J, King R and O'Brien T (2019) The Peer Supervision Group as Clinical Research Device: Analysis of a Group Experience. *British Journal of Psychotherapy*, 35 (2): 305–321.

Yerushalmi H (1999) The Roles of Group Supervision of Supervision. *Psychoanalytic Psychology*, 16 (3): 426–447.

Chapter 13

Using the Group as a Medium of Supervision

Amelie Noack

Introduction

Supervision is now firmly acknowledged as one of the three cornerstones of analytic training alongside theory and personal analysis. Good supervision provides a safe container and enables thinking, models competence and contributes to the development of a professional identity. Supervisors may assess a candidate's readiness for qualification, but generally offer observation, support, education and challenge, as well as knowledge of theory, practice and ethics. In any good supervision the unconscious meaning of the communications between patient and therapist will emerge more clearly and the supervisee's ability to recognise the importance of transference and countertransference processes will develop as well as their capacity to handle them.

The value of group supervision

While trainees are required to be in supervision, experienced practitioners also use supervision to gain from the supervisor's external viewpoint of the therapeutic relationship(s)—this also brings triangulation into play. Group analysts in general continue in supervision after training, whether with a senior colleague or with peers, to find 'the third eye' (Sharpe, 1995), which is necessary in view of the complex dynamics in groups. Individual therapists working with more disturbed, perverse or violent patients are also in particular need of a containing space for thinking to counterbalance the attacks on the therapist's mind inherent in this taxing kind of work (Bion, 1984). These supervisory relationships, which are often established after training and after ending personal therapeutic work, require additional skills from the supervisor. Continuing sometimes for years, for the practitioner the relationship with the supervisor often becomes the closest personal attachment in the matrix of professional relationships. In such work the supervisor will have to learn to work not only with the supervised patient's material, but also with the personal material of the supervisee, and they will need to develop an especially sensitive approach to deciding when to address this. While it would be useful to expand on this aspect, this is, regrettably, beyond the remit of this chapter.

DOI: 10.4324/9781032719085-17

My expertise and experience as a supervisor over many years was originally based on the individual psychoanalytical model and a supervisors' training course. Having since undergone training in group analysis at the Institute of Group Analysis in London, as well as a group analytic supervision course, my understanding of the supervisory process has considerably grown. I want to use this opportunity to reflect on the change in my supervisory attitude and practice due to the group analytic input. Group analytic-orientated supervision relies to a certain extent on the same psychoanalytical theories and principles as individual supervision, such as transference and counter-transference dynamics, projective identification and the like. However, groups present a more complex phenomenon than the dyadic patient-therapist situation and require additional concepts and skills. The group analytic model and a group analytic viewpoint provide the necessary means to accommodate, understand and handle this complexity.

Some complexities of group supervision

Yalom emphasises the *complexity* of working with groups, when he states that supervision of group therapy is more taxing than individual supervision, and this is not only because there could be approximately eight people in each group to keep in mind (Yalom, 1995). This may well be true. My aim here, however, is not to focus on the difficulties of supervising groups, since this topic has been well explored in *The Third Eye* (Sharpe, 1995). Here, I would like to describe some group analytic concepts and some tools group analysis has developed to deal with the inherent complexity of working with groups and apply them to supervision in general. The group analytic viewpoint will, I hope, add to the scope and understanding of processes occurring in supervision.

One of the main differences between group and individual work is the fact that group analysis emphasises that part of therapeutic work belonging to frame, setting and management by using its own name, 'dynamic administration'. Trainees and newly qualified therapists are usually so eager to do what they consider the 'proper work' of a therapist, namely interpreting, that they may neglect the more basic tasks of the therapist. Dynamic administration focuses on the establishment of a secure 'holding environment' and a working alliance with the patient, as well as the maintenance of boundaries, and makes it clear that there exists an immutable division with clear boundaries between the work done inside and outside of the group. This in turn provides the group with a secure space for psychic exploration. I consider holding, the working alliance and boundaries, the groundwork of any therapeutic activity. The group analytic focus on dynamic administration allows the supervisor to highlight the importance of the establishment of these basic aspects, and to point out that they are solely the responsibility of the therapist. If this is overlooked, dropouts or negative therapeutic reactions may follow.

In the domain of dynamic administration, the group analyst reigns supreme and may even be seen as dictatorial. This is complemented and balanced by the advantages of the democratic process of the group analytic method since, in the therapeutic process within the group, agency is shared by the facilitator with the group. This means in practice that every group member is in the same position as the therapist to make observations, which might be succinct and fitting interpretations of what is going on in the group at the time. This approach makes use of the strengths of the multi-perspective aspect of the group and, combined with the increasing capacity for insight, facilitates a sense of synergy through difference, while establishing at the same time a sense of similarity through understanding.

The group analytic principle of *resonance*, which has an impact on each group member and on the group as a whole, evokes free association, which in the group takes the form of shared dialogue and discourse. Sooner or later this develops into *free group discussion* and in time the deepening aspects of free group discussion take over the role of traditional psychoanalytical interpretation. The complementary working together of both these aspects, dynamic administration and shared therapeutic work, and the understanding that these are overlapping processes taking place at the same time, contribute to the group analytic attitude. A supervisor with a group analytic attitude will hold these different aspects in mind, as well as facilitate the involvement of all the supervisees in the supervisory process to enable them to make their own contributions and also learn from the others. Foulkes, the founder of group analysis, called this process *ego-training in action* in parallel to the constructive process of ego-building in the traditional psychoanalytic model of individual therapy (Foulkes, 1964: 74).

In addition to the holding frame and boundaries, the supervisor has to pay attention to the interactions in the supervision group. *Group dynamics* may manifest in a variety of ways in supervision groups, and Fuller and Scanlon, among others, have described how the dynamics of Bion's basic assumption attitudes are displayed in supervision groups (Fuller, 2003; Scanlon, 2002). I would like to mention two further dynamic situations that occur in supervision and manifest either on a vertical or a horizontal plane. Between members of a supervision group, conscious or unconscious competition, rivalry and envy might appear. Similar issues may also emerge among professionals and become evident in committee work, combined with status and rank concerns. An awareness of this is often suppressed, since nobody wants to become the scapegoat. These phenomena, described by Parker and Wilke, usually materialise on a horizontal level and demonstrate sibling dynamics (Parker, 2020; Wilke, 2014). They need to be understood as such and hopefully can be talked through in the supervision group to make people conscious of these dynamics. In addition to the conflictual feelings between equals or peers, dynamics in a supervision group may also manifest in relation to authority. For instance, profound anxiety or inability about presenting one's work in supervision, idealisation or severe critique of the supervisor's technique or attitude, or provocative boundary transgressions, like arriving late or asking for extra time, would indicate problems with authority and are related to the supervisor's position. These issues demonstrate the power dynamics on the vertical plane and also need to be understood and appropriately addressed. It is the supervisor's role to grasp the nettle and tackle these issues in the supervision group. It is not an easy task, especially if it concerns the supervisor's own personality.

Both these dynamics of conflict on the horizontal or vertical axis within the supervision group illustrate some of the more complicated, possibly destructive, or even aggressive and potentially traumatic experiences, which may emerge and might be acted out in the supervisory group. What transpires may well be derived from the respective patients' dynamics, and the group analytic concepts of *resonance* and *mirroring* highlight what of the individual or group under discussion may be reflected in the supervision group. *Resonance* and *mirroring* are two group analytic concepts that describe the parallel process, a notion going back to Searles' idea of the reflective process (Searles, 1955). While Zinkin asserts that what happens in therapy is unique and ultimately incommunicable, the participants in the supervisory space can get a glimpse of the interactions in the therapeutic space through using the parallel process (Zinkin, 1995). A well-functioning supervision group reproduces a reaction to the material under supervision, which usually is a fair reflection of the state of the individual or group presented by the supervisee. For instance, a rather helpless atmosphere in the supervision group would indicate helplessness in the therapeutic space. This may well have been experienced by the group during the particular session where it is being presented. Supervision can then serve to initiate the process of mentalisation for split-off or encapsulated psychic parts by holding them in the supervisory space and contemplating the events, so they can begin to be thought about.

Using the group as a medium for supervision

When using the group as a medium of supervision, it is essential to use the full potential of the supervision group. This works best when supervision reflects the fundamental value system of group analysis and includes the importance of principles like *mutuality* and *interdependence*. Group analysis stresses that the therapeutic process in a group is 'analysis of the group, by the group including the conductor' (Foulkes, 1964: 3). This describes the fact that group members as well as the conductor are all equally exposed to the impact of events occurring in the *matrix* of the group during the session. While it is well known that a patient's developmental process occurs in correlation to the practitioner's capacity for change and further development, working as a group analyst throws this notion into further relief.

As the group conductor I am more exposed to the impact of events in the session than an individual analyst, because I am not sitting behind the couch, but in a circle on the same kind of chair as everybody else, visible to each and everyone. My own resistances or defences may to a certain degree be visible in a similar way to those of every other group member. This visibility is usually also distorted by transferences, but the group is always there to offer a corrective to that. It is often exposure and shame that patients fear from therapy and, as a group conductor, I find myself in a similarly vulnerable position. This is a sobering experience and constantly forces me to reassess the function of shame and exposure in therapy and, consequently, in supervision.

Some group analytic language

The complexity of communications and events in each group session can at times feel overwhelming. This might be due to projective identifications, which may attack the therapist's capacity for thought, but there are also other occasions, when resonances reverberate within the group and associations are amplified and assembled, resulting in the group analytic *condenser phenomenon*. These are moments when the group analyst must be able to tolerate 'not knowing' and remember Foulkes' notion of 'trusting the group'. Condenser phenomena are events in which the therapeutic or supervisory process may move on to a new level of understanding or meaning, akin to the notion of a quantum leap in physics.

The capacity to stay with 'not knowing' may be difficult, but it is essential for any meaningful therapeutic activity, and this includes supervision. The capacity of learning to tolerate 'not knowing' means to develop what Keats called 'negative capability'. This is being able to tolerate 'being in uncertainties, mysteries, doubts, without any irritable reaching after fact & reason' (Keats, 1817). Within this space, which I consider akin to Bion's notion of 'O' (Bion, 1965; Bion, 1970), creativity and transformation can come into being, and out of this space new meaning may emerge. This applies, I believe, to therapy as well as supervision. If the group conductor or supervisor can manage these difficult moments of 'not knowing' and work under such conditions, which means to be able to maintain or in time recapture the capacity to think, the supervisees and patients will eventually also learn to do the same.

The ability to identify this space of 'not knowing' and differentiate it from resistance or defensiveness, presupposes the conductor's or the supervisor's aptitude for *translation*, another group analytic concept that I find especially useful. In addition to the psychoanalytic concept of interpretation, Foulkes introduced the notion of translation, through which meaning is traced and defined (Foulkes, 1964: 66). Translations are the group analytic equivalent to making the unconscious conscious. They are verbal communications by members of the group, which convert primary process into secondary process language or move the symptomatic on to the symbolic level of thinking and understanding. They can take various verbal forms, like drawing attention to something, linking, confronting or interpreting. Translation is an essential part of communication, given that every individual—and every group for that matter—has their own specific language or idiom. In therapeutic work we are always translating the patients' language into our own and vice versa, and supervision has to juggle additional translation processes, which are propounded in group supervision.

Conclusion

In conclusion I would like to mention the importance that group analysis places on the *social dimension* and on the notions of *mutuality* and *interdependence*, ideas and concepts that all take an underlying shared human matrix for granted. Foulkes referred to Jung's idea of the collective unconscious, when describing his idea of the foundation matrix in groups. The concept of the foundation matrix points to a shared understanding between Jungian thinking and the thinking of group analysis in regard to the notion of a fundamental layer of psychic life that encompasses individual and collective processes: '...just as the individual is not unique and separate, but is also a social being, so the human psyche is not a self-contained and wholly individual phenomenon, but also a collective one' (Jung, 1977: 144).

In the Western world, we usually consider the individual as the originator of thought and thinking. The thought of all life, including being human, as an interdependent whole may well be experienced as intolerable since, for many people, the idea of mutual dependence is a frightening notion. Therefore, Western thought tends to deny the importance of a joint human matrix as the basis of all relationships and all thought. In contrast, the group analytic concept of a matrix of interdependent and mutual relationships takes account of individual as well as collective and social phenomena. It accepts the dynamic notion of a socially grounded individual within a shared human matrix, and this view offers the basis for a new psychotherapeutic paradigm. If engaging in supervision helps us to develop a 'third eye', which offers triangulation as a new viewpoint, group analytic supervision might be trying to push the development one step further. It might open the way for a new way of lateral seeing, where we may be able, eventually, to allow for a many-sided or multifaceted point of view. This would presuppose, however, the ability to truly tolerate difference and diversity.

References

Bion W (1965) *Transformations*. Karnac Books.
Bion W (1970) *Attention and Interpretation*. Karnac Books.

Bion W (1984) *Second Thoughts*. Karnac Books.

Foulkes SH (1964) *Therapeutic Group Analysis*. Allen & Unwin. (Reprinted 1984: Karnac Books.)

Fuller VG (2003) *Supervision in Groups*. In: Wiener J, Mizen R and Duckham J (eds), *Supervising and Being Supervised*. Palgrave Macmillan.

Jung CG (1977) *Two Essays on Analytical Psychology. Collected Works*, Volume 7. Princeton University Press.

Keats J (1817) Letter to his brothers of 21 Dec 1817. In: www.geocities.com/Athens/Parthenon/4942/negcap.html.

Parker V (2020) *A Group-Analytic Exploration of the Sibling Matrix: How Siblings Shape our Lives*. Routledge.

Scanlon C (2002) Group Supervision of Individual Cases in the Training of Counsellors and Psychotherapists: Towards a Group-Analytic Model? *British Journal of Psychotherapy*, 19 (2): 219–235.

Searles HF (1955) The Informational Value of the Supervisor's Emotional Experience. In: *Collected Papers on Schizophrenia and Related Subjects*. Karnac Books.

Sharpe M (ed.) (1995) *The Third Eye: Supervision of Analytic Groups*. Routledge.

Wilke G (2014) *The Art of Group Analysis in Organisations: The Use of Intuitive and Experiential Knowledge*. Karnac Books.

Yalom I (1995) *The Theory and Practice of Group Psychotherapy*. Basic Books.

Zinkin L (1995) *Supervision: The Impossible Profession*. In: Kugler P (ed.), *Jungian Perspectives on Clinical Supervision*. Daimon.

Part 5

Ethics and Group Supervision

Chapter 14

Is Group Supervision Ethical?

Frances Griffiths

Introduction

Ethics comes from the Greek for ethos meaning character. The *Oxford English Dictionary* suggests a simple definition: 'the discipline concerned with what is morally good and bad and morally right and wrong'.

> By their very nature ethics are not absolutes. They change as the cultural and scientific evidence demands.
>
> (Behr and Hearst, 2005: 249)

This somewhat provocative assertion, and the recent experience of the seismic cultural rupture of COVID 19, focuses our minds on the question of group supervision as ethical. Never before had we experienced the impact of a global pandemic that necessitated an unexpected and urgent response as to how to rethink how we conduct our training, clinical practice and supervision. Creating an ethical framework around the move to online sessions created many opportunities and many challenges. The benefits expressed by those who do not wish to return to face-to-face supervision sessions include the time and money saved by *not* having to travel, justified in a culture of a growing wealth divide; not necessarily having to negotiate the obstacles demanded by being disabled and/or ageing; and the ability to conduct a group with members not in the immediate location. These might be thought of as ethical solutions in a changing culture. However, these seemingly obvious solutions present new challenges and raise questions about what we might call 'practical ethics'. The emergence of ordinary conversations about how we are seen and appear in virtual reality has led to many more questions.

What is ethical when one is in virtual contact with clients and supervisees? Is it acceptable for supervisees to see you in a setting other than the usual one of your consulting room? Perhaps even more unusually we (supervisor and supervisees) have been allowed into each other's living spaces. Over the past four years I have seen supervisees in their cars (the only way to ensure a confidential space when one is sharing a house), in a hotel room (when one

DOI: 10.4324/9781032719085-19

supervisee had arrived suddenly as a migrant from overseas), and in the garden (when the weather permitted). Additionally, I have spoken with clients who did not have access to technology and preferred to speak on the phone.

This sudden rupture from in-person supervision with the whole bodies of supervisees and supervisor in the same room, while creating something of a dilemma for the regulatory framework, has perhaps created a more egalitarian opportunity for us as supervisors. These opportunities come in the form of questions that I see as the lifeblood of ethics and ethical practice. The importance of questioning all that we do is at the centre of an ethical framework and this global event has stimulated the need for us to question our supervision practice as ethical.

There is much to be thought about here in the context of change and the dilemma posed by ethics not being about absolutes, exemplified for example by the question of confidentiality. The regulatory framework expects us to observe client confidentiality. Is this an absolute? If so, can our practice be considered ethical? The regulatory framework stresses the importance of supervision for keeping ourselves and the supervisees safe, and yet we cast aside absolute confidentiality when we bring our work to supervision. Is this a boundary violation, or an example of ethical safeguarding and good practice? This is just one dilemma, for, if ethics is all about non-absolutes, how do we navigate what seems to be an absolute. In the 'best interests of clients' we are told, 'not (to) have sexual contact or sexual relationships with clients' (UKCP, 2019: 4:1).[1] We all agree on the importance of this imperative, or do we? What challenges do these situations pose to our internal ethical supervisor (Casement, 1985) and to the regulatory framework?

There are other situations which are not as clear-cut, and it could be that 'ethics that are not absolutes' provoke the most fear and anxiety. For example, ageing, migration, sudden illness and disability and a growing wealth gap are not clear-cut in themselves. In such a case a resort to a hierarchy of values intervenes at a conscious level to influence the choices we make. However, in the realm of the unconscious we require the eyes and ears of the group to help us to think and pose new questions. This is what might be thought of as ethical, for everything is worth noticing and it is in the spirit of enquiry about our practice and the framework that we co-create that ensures it is ethical. In this way we develop a 'third eye' (Sharpe, 1995). It is in the process of often seemingly ordinary conversations in supervision that the thinking process is given space to do its work of giving thought to new ways of thinking. It is this circular reflexive activity that creates a solid and safe foundation in and on which to develop moral courage, as the following vignette demonstrates. My experience as a trainee led me to question my awareness of the threat to ethical practice if turning a blind eye and a deaf ear were the cultural norm.

Vignette: The experience of a trainee group analyst

Many years ago, as a trainee group analyst, I was on placement in a large NHS outpatient department offering a range of therapeutic modalities to adult patients. In this setting a large group supervision session was held weekly so that, over a number of weeks, each trainee in turn could present their dyadic patient-therapist session to a range of experienced therapists and novice trainees. It was a very valuable learning experience but, oddly, as a trainee group analyst I was not included on this roster. There seemed to be the thought that a group session would be too difficult to present. Perhaps I held on to the fear that this large group would be unable to make sense of there being several people in the consulting room at the same time. For a long time, I sat and listened observing the dynamics of relationships in this setting as they constellated around those who seemingly knew and those who did not know what was going on. It had the capacity to be deeply shaming if one got it wrong. Eventually I proposed presenting my training therapy group in one of these supervision sessions.

The response was interesting and inspiring. The whole group, experienced and trainee therapists became involved in relating to the group members and the material. The emphasis was not on the group conductor, me, and what I was doing or not doing, but on the supervision group as they busied themselves in the parallel process of relating to the session. The group therapy session had included the metaphor of a cake, enabling us to think about the space and time available. It was felt by one member that she only got the crumbs while others seemed to take more than they might have needed. The large group supervision mirrored the therapy group. Some people took up huge amounts of space and time, not appearing to notice they had had more than their share. Eventually the time and space to think about what was going on in the supervision group opened up sufficiently for almost everyone to find a voice, just as I had found my voice. Co-creation appeared in the language of reciprocity and mutuality. I began to appreciate the importance of the parallel process and so much more. Amplification and resonance supported my growing confidence in the ethics of group supervision. Many eyes and ears, hearts and minds helped me over many weeks to see and hear blind spots, to develop an appreciation of the parallel process and a thirst to undertake group analytic supervision training—and many years later to my interest in ethics and ethical practice.

My interest in group supervision as ethical, while very present and important, creates something of a dilemma. It is this dilemma that I suggest lies at the heart of our practice. As group supervisors and supervisees, we might think the notion that important issues are always obvious, and we pay attention to them. The evidence suggests otherwise, and we may all have had experience of not having noticed the seemingly glaringly obvious. In the consulting room we think about the work of supervision through the widest possible lens but what happens when there are 'blind spots and new challenges' such as those presented by Covid? How do we set about addressing the demands of cultural developments and scientific evidence and detect bias? A well-functioning supervision group will be open and aware of looking out for conscious and unconscious bias in every area. 'Reciprocity and mutuality' will be present in the supervision group as it works to create a shared language, which is not fully understood or shared (Dalal, 2021: 18). The legalistic language is not the language of the clinic, and this creates a problem. Or does it? This is at the heart of my dilemma and mirrors a dilemma for organisations.

This experience exemplifies the dilemma for clinicians when the organisation/institution turns a 'blind eye' to the inclusion of group analytic supervision. I had been blinded by the culture of an institute wedded to a dyadic way of working in supervision. Importantly, it stressed how an institution shapes our way of thinking, for it revealed the power of a predetermined cultural perspective of an institute with a common shared belief and investment in working in a dyadic way. It took some time for me to challenge this status quo and to open my eyes to the power of the mirroring effect of a 'blind spot' that existed in me, the group and the institute. A 'blind spot' that had annihilated a space in terms of the benefits of what we could do as a whole supervision group. The benefits of an ongoing conversation in the group analytic tradition offers the opportunity 'to learn something new [and] entails changing one's whole attitude to a number of things, to "oneself" and to the world in which one lives' (Foulkes, 1990: 224–225). This is profound and there is more to write about this phenomenon. I believe it demonstrates in a powerful manner the importance of inclusion of the whole group as an ethical dimension of our practice.

To return to my dilemma. I am in the position of wearing two hats. One is as a group analytic clinician and supervisor, and the other is as chair of the ethics committee of the College of Psychoanalytic and Jungian Analysts (CPJA). My immediate experience as ethics chair is that responsibility for ethics is often understood to reside at the organisational level of the membership organisation and accrediting organisation, UKCP. As chair of the ethics committee, it may be that I am seen as judge and jury of ethical practice as if I am the expert on ethics. This would be to grossly overestimate my role, and also to detract from the responsibility we each have as practitioners for our own awareness of our ethical practices and for safeguarding. This might seem daunting when seen in terms of the legalistic language of UKCP Guidelines.

This language might be seen as beyond comprehension when ethics becomes all about complaints and grievance procedures. However, in my view this is a reductionist approach that leaves little space for thinking. Instead, ethics and ethical practice invite us to engage in a lively discussion about the boundaries around our everyday relationships. But there is a caveat here.

'Careful reflection and reflexive practice' require our constant attention to the language, spoken and unspoken in group supervision, in the process of which we awaken to the possibility of blind spots that blur our vision, obscuring the dilemmas of everyday practice about what is morally good and bad, and right and wrong. This necessitates our constant attention that begins with acknowledging the fear that the regulatory framework imposes and the importance of supervision and supervision training that mitigates this fear. This then brings into focus further questions about how we use our power and authority as supervisors and supervisees and leads to an exploration of 'moral courage'. As a practitioner I question how I can become familiar with a benign authority at the bedrock of an ethical way of being in myself and in the group. I start with understanding the fear, attributed mostly to the regulatory framework that threatens to destabilise this bedrock.

Fear of the regulatory framework

When asked, 'What is the most important issue facing supervision today?' Shohet replied, 'To realise how much fear there is in our work' (Shohet, 2022). As chair of the ethics committee, I am witness to the anxiety caused when there is a misunderstanding and/or a misinterpretation of the language of the legal framework. Sometimes the fear of litigation, which appears to be at the heart of the anxiety, stifles the capacity to think and question what we do and a slavish adherence to the language of regulation often appears at odds with the language and practice in the clinic, which is exploratory and exists in a culture of 'not knowing' (Keats, 1817). An exploration of the language we use to describe the supervisory relationship, by its very nature fraught with the certainty of misunderstandings and misinterpretations, can lead to new ways of thinking and being.

This is to be welcomed in an increasingly overregulated world. The stimulating dialogue questioning the issue of power in the supervisory relationship as seen in the recent exchange between Dalal (2021) and Bacha (2023) is the basis of a firm foundation on which to build an ethical practice. In this lively and engaging dialogue, they disagree about the nature of the supervisory relationship in which they each see things differently. Bacha sees it as an unequal relationship in which power is always present. Dalal does not deny the absence of power in the relationship. He sees power as, 'ever present', while asserting the language of reciprocity and mutuality in the supervisory relationship are necessary for it to be deemed ethical. The subject of power appears central in their disagreement, while Bacha proposes that the difficulty they may have is understanding each other's use of language, which includes differences 'in' and 'of' supervision.

This discussion will hopefully be picked up by others. If the issue is that of unequal power relations co-created in the supervision space between therapist and supervisor, we might anticipate the presence of considerable anxiety and an unwillingness to question the status quo. Is your supervisor up to the mark? Do they observe agreed boundaries? Is the supervisee able to present a therapy that enables others to question and engage in a lively discussion about the work? Are they able to let their vulnerability be seen and heard? For, somewhat perversely, it is in being vulnerable that power resides—not absolute power but non-malignant power that allows for an internal reconfiguration, a recalibration of one's values and morals.

We need more lively dialogues such as this to lift ethics off the page and bring it to the foreground of our practice. It is central to who we are, but it questions how we create the space for thought as to how and, if need be, to make sense of two different languages. This is pertinent in the face of the creeping bureaucratisation of our practice as supervisors. One of the challenges, however, is how to satisfy these demands.

My experience for the past four years as chair of the ethics committee (CPJA) and as a practising group analytic supervisor has helped me to think about how to marry two different languages and question whether this is possible. This thorny issue impacts our practice. It immediately puts me at the heart of a dilemma that introduces the notion of a hierarchy of power relations in which the regulatory function might be perceived as being above, more important than, our clinical experience—as if, for example, we fear inadvertently finding ourselves involved in a dispute about ethical boundaries. This is a real issue and one that I feel requires more attention to the regulatory framework, which is there to be worked with and not feared.

A further dilemma is a somewhat legalistic one. It has to do with hierarchy and is beyond the scope of this chapter, but points to an unresolved situation in the relationship of two UKCP documents that do not appear to stand together seamlessly. At present, for example, the UKCP Code of Ethics and Professional Practice appears to be the final arbiter in a court of law with regard to our clinical practice, with an established complaints and appeals process. However, the UKCP Practice Guidelines for Supervisors has no such complaints or appeals process (UKCP, 2018). It is perhaps a moot point as to whether the absence of a supervision complaints and appeals process weakens the defence of it as ethical practice. It raises the question, 'Can we, however, justify and validate our practice as ethical when there is an absence of a complaints and appeals process against a supervisor?'. This is currently the subject of much discussion at the College of Psychoanalytic and Jungian Association executive meetings.

Do we as practitioners make links and keep in mind the demands of two different languages: one that takes account of morals and values in the psychotherapeutic endeavour of working with the unconscious; the other that is enshrined in a Code of Ethics and Professional Practice that impacts on our practice (UKCP, 2019)? I believe we can by getting to know the codes that might contain ambiguities that can be challenged.

The UKCP 2019 code states, 'Ensure [that] you are familiar and understand the UKCP's published policies', 'Challenge questionable practice in yourself and others' and '[Ensure] continuing ability to practise by securing supervision and ongoing professional education and development sufficient to meet the requirements of UKCP, its modality colleges and its organisational members' (UKCP, 2019: 25).

This appears to reinforce the important place of supervision in minding the boundaries around ethical practice. Does it take the fear out of the regulatory framework?

Taking the fear out of the regulatory framework

The fear of the regulatory function appears to be based on the premise that the language of the clinic stands in contradiction to a more legalistic language that is seen as absolute. While this is partly true, it is also the case that the UKCP Practice Guidelines for Supervisors (2018) is written in everyday language that we can understand and we can agree with. It says, 'Supervision is understood as a process conducted within a formal working relationship' (1.5), 'in which a Psychotherapeutic Practitioner or Trainee presents their clinical work to a designated supervisor as a way of enhancing their practice through careful reflection and reflexive practice on the process' (UKCP, 2018: 2.1, p. 3) and, 'Supervision can take place in facilitated groups, peer groups' and that 'Appropriate modes of supervision will need to be determined by the circumstances' (UKCP, 2018: 2.2, p. 3). This suggests that supervision allows for situations that are not absolutes; and it promotes; 'Supervision [that] should perform the functions of education, support and evaluation *against* the norms and standards of the modality, profession and society' (UKCP, 2018: 3.2, p. 3).

What is stressed in the Guidelines is the importance of supervision and, importantly, the above extracts from the Guidelines suggest the need for supervision training. However, what the literature seems to suggest is that there is an absence of attention to ethics and ethical practice in the culture of supervision training.

Ethics and training

There is evidence in the literature of the importance of supervision training but also of the absence of ethics as a part of the training. Barnett noted 'Training courses have neglected this area [of ethic]) in the past', and proposed that therapists need to know the law with regard to professional practice, including keeping up to date with any recent changes. Somewhat strongly she proposed, 'There is much fear surrounding supervisors and therapists being caught in litigation and how therapeutic language may be misconstrued in the legal process' (Barnett, 2005: 154, 152).

Sharpe warns of the dangers of complacency. She suggests complacency is the enemy and that it is 'constant alertness' and peer supervision that can serve to protect us. Covering 11 training areas in total, she stressed the centrality of ethics, which can offset legal challenges, explaining that these arise from legal liabilities of supervisor and institution. Sharpe justified training of supervisors on many grounds, one of which was uniformity of training and experience act as a protective framework against litigation. She makes reference to 'ethics and personal integrity' as 'An area of great sensitivity and importance to a fully professional supervisor' (Sharpe, 1995: 160).

Meg Sharpe's seminal work on the practice of group supervision continues to be as important today as it was when written in 1995. Inculcating a 'third eye' is made possible by the number of eyes looking at the dilemma in the supervision group. Dimensions of difference from every view are made possible in a group supervision space of a diverse group of members prepared to listen with a third ear, paying attention to what is being said, prepared and ready to think and to question every aspect. Resonance and amplification have a place, and cohesion is guarded against by spotting it as a possible obstacle, a defence in the face of coherence. The importance of this work is taken further by Smith and Gallop who build on this earlier work to develop a theoretical framework of group analytic supervision training, as in their year-long training at the Institute of Group Analysis (Smith and Gallop, 2023).

Smith and Gallop draw attention in their recent book, *Group Analytic Supervision* to the importance of training gaps and changing cultural norms in the areas of 'ethics, diversity and intersectionality, endings and retirements, student perspective and organisational issues' (Smith and Gallop, 2023: 4). They suggest there is further work needed in these areas to create a space in which to think about the ethical impact of these cultural developments on our supervisory relationships.

Congruence and moral courage to address issues

Congruence can be thought of as equivalence (Griffiths, 2023) in the structure of the group's tripartite matrix (foundation, dynamic and the personal) (Hopper, 2023), in which the concept of the social unconscious and thinking is key. The power of the group analytic supervision process lies in the creation of a space in which many eyes and many ears are devoted to looking for congruence. However, congruence co-exists with incongruence, and it is the co-existence of this dual relationship that presents an opportunity for the dynamic encounter in the supervision group that enables it to resist complacency. However, the seduction of the 'simple solution' approach has cultural currency in the present climate, and this makes group supervision all the more important and necessary.

A current cultural norm can be seen at the level of the foundation, dynamic and personal matrix of organisations in the fields of politics, business, education and sport (and there may be other examples). An accolade for success co-exists in the matrix with the fear of failure and demotion for the organisation and those in it, as if they count for nothing. We see how this plays out at every level. Examples include football managers who have been fired just because their team loses and the team is demoted in the league tables. Within education, schools can be castigated as 'failing', based on pupil achievement and 'safeguarding', without taking full account of levels of deprivation. This can lead to burnout and in some cases, headteachers and teachers leave. Politicians and the electorate demand a change of leader when opinion polls dip. Scapegoating is often seen as a solution in the face of something else that is overlooked. All organisations including psychotherapy networks and training can fall prey to scapegoating without proper attention paid to the importance of supervision and calling things out. Standing up to the abuse of power that often exists at the highest level requires moral courage at every level.

The courage to say when something does not feel right and when there is the need for more thought is often complicated by the nature of the relationship. In psychotherapy training organisations, it may not be easy for a supervisee to point out that the supervisory relationship is unsatisfactory. The supervisor may not always keep abreast of cultural changes and a supervisee pointing this out may not have the required effect of asking the group to think about this dilemma. However, in the face of change, thinking is key, and this is *always* the case as Behr and Hearst suggest (2005). There will always be the need to meet the demands of cultural change and scientific evidence, and the COVID epidemic is an example and an opportunity to put into context the impact on our moral values in response to sudden change. Change can unblock and make visible things we have previously not seen and, according to Tubert-Oklander, this can happen when 'there is a rupture, a commotion, or catastrophe in the sociopolitical context that both analyst and group members or patients share ... meaning a situation in which the members and the conductor are "together in the same boat", under the impact of the shared social trauma, and must also work it through together' (Tubert-Oklander, 2018: 80).

I. Disability and sudden illness

A vivid and contemporaneous example of a social trauma that necessitated unexpected and immediate changes to our practices resides in the case of the recent global pandemic, COVID-19. The impact of this social trauma was felt at many levels and, for the first time ever, we experienced the feeling of all being 'in the same boat', although of course we were *not* all in the same boat, as history has revealed. For some, adaptation to online virtual ways of working in a secure environment with a healthy bank balance and the introduction of free COVID vaccinations has meant that life could go on fairly smoothly. The imposition of sudden change could be managed reasonably equitably and for some the changes were welcomed. However, for others' lives were changed forever. The impact of having caught COVID and the consequences for some of having long COVID have parallels with being affected by the unexpected diagnosis of illness and/or disability. Everyone else may have a choice as to how and which adaptations suit their circumstances. However, for those suddenly diagnosed with a long-term crippling illness, requiring painful physical treatment, there may not be a choice. In this situation as in the case with a supervisee in a group I supervised, we had to think about how to manage this situation.

The supervisee in training had been planning, with the support of the supervision group, to take on a first patient case. The timing appeared appropriate, and the supervision group had expressed their interest in the trainee's patient that had been brought to the group over a number of weeks in preparation for an agreed start date. Without any warning the supervisee began to feel unwell and a resistance to thinking about this as anything other than a natural response to the anxiety of taking on their first patient created a 'blind eye' to what else might be going on. When eventually the supervisee was encouraged to see a medical practitioner, it transpired there was indeed a good reason for them feeling unwell. The devastating diagnosis and the feeling in the group of guilt and shame over having seemingly turned a 'blind eye' and a 'deaf ear' to hearing what was being said threatened the ethical boundaries of the group. Could it be a safe place? What had we missed? Could we contain this difficult and challenging situation?

2. Ageing

I think one of the most difficult dilemmas we each face is when and how to end our professional work with which we are engaged. In many other occupations there is an age by which one is expected to retire. However, in private practice as a psychotherapist and supervisor there is no upper age limit, and we can go on for much longer—sometimes until we drop. This is a very serious issue.

The dilemma is how to think as an individual, a group and an organisation about age and ageing and retiring. The medical profession has adopted a 'duty of candour' meaning the professional members have a duty to take care of each other in the interests of the patient, the team and the reputation of the profession. There is nothing as yet in the psychotherapy codes to help us with this dilemma and yet there may have been incidences where this could have safeguarded the therapist, the client and the organisation. Indeed, SH Foulkes, credited with being the father of group analysis in the UK, died while conducting a group. One would imagine the responsibility each of us has, for example, for a group supervision group would demand that we take care of each other. The dilemma is how we go about this delicate issue. Do we tap a colleague on the shoulder and suggest an informal discussion to think about what has been observed. Or do we turn a blind eye expecting someone else to do this on our behalf.

One therapist, when asked when she might retire, said, 'I keep on working in order to stave off my inevitable demise. I work to keep death at bay'. We should ask, 'Is this ethical?', but my observation suggests we turn a 'blind eye' to ageing. What is the reluctance to give thought to the process of ageing, when to give up and how to encourage others to see this an opportunity. An opportunity to offer a life time's wealth of experience in the support of those just embarking on a training course for whom the current ethical challenges are many and changing all the time.

3. Wealth gap

During the recent pandemic when the world was so disrupted, many lost their sources of income and were unsure how to pay for supervision. This has proved to be the situation in which many have found themselves. The challenge has been to temper one's financial expectations as a supervisor in order to meet the requirements of a supervisee in recognition that we have a great deal to learn from each other. Learning is the quid pro quo of our profession. Generosity is key.

There may be a further ethical dilemma for trainees who may not want to let their supervisor know that they have financial difficulties because of changing circumstances. In a recent case, a supervisor on a training course with a number of trainees in their group knew of the strained circumstances of a supervisee but failed to acknowledge it on the grounds that it would undermine cohesion and equality. If the supervisee were to pay a lesser amount how would the others in the group feel about this? In addition, the supervisor had bills to pay like everyone else, a lifestyle and a reputation to protect. This situation was resolved when the supervisee left the group and found a supervisor who charged a lower fee. Might this have been avoided by thinking about it ethically?

4. Migration

Contemporaneous changes in the demographics of our world of psychotherapy practice mirror many of the global problems we see about us today. They also parallel the challenge of making sense of two different language and cultural dimensions of the regulatory framework and our clinical work. The meaning can sometimes be lost in translation as we have seen. Oversights and blind sight create a challenge to our ethical practices and to our relationships. There are parallels here.

We sometimes turn a blind eye to the language of the ethical guidelines for fear of not understanding the language. We may defend against this fear by refusing to acknowledge the importance of what they offer us. We may do the same with a member of the group who, having suddenly migrated to a new country, as is the case with some practitioners from Ukraine and Russia, is adapting to a new culture, a new language and a new frame of reference. In a culture of humility how do we make sense of their experience and acknowledge the opportunity we have to learn from each other. Central to this pursuit are the *relationships* we co-create and what counts as ethical. The question of the relationships we create and the challenge to understand each other is paramount as the dialogue between two experienced group analysts and supervisors shows: Dalal proposes two important elements that validate the supervisory encounter as ethical while also acknowledging the existence of a power dynamic that is always present in the clinic. This power dynamic is recognised in the regulatory guidance as a warning. I believe it is this understanding that brings the two ethical languages of the clinic and the legal eagles together in a relationship that is understood and shared by both partners.

Supervisory relationships

Reciprocity and mutuality

Dalal asserts the co-creation of a relationship in which reciprocity and mutuality are evident makes it ethical (Dalal, 2021). Bacha (2021) profoundly disagrees with Dalal. For Bacha, 'Supervisory relationships are generally defined as unequal in power and authority' and therefore supervision relationships can never be deemed mutual and reciprocal. Dalal (2022) replies that he experienced neither in a recent supervisory relationship, to which Bacha responds that for Dalal an absence of reciprocity and mutuality makes a supervisory relationship unethical (Bacha, 2021: 94).

It is important to understand what Dalal means by reciprocity and mutuality. In his response to the challenge posited by Bacha that reciprocity and mutuality in the supervisory relationship overlooks issues of power and authority, he refutes this view. For Dalal, reciprocity 'keeps in mind the ever-present power relations between supervisor and supervisee' (Dalal, 2021: 16). This is what is at the heart of the co-creation of mutuality in the group. It is, he asserts, this process that makes supervision ethical. The disagreement between these two group analysts 'on the level of his definition of relational' tells us a great deal about the space for misunderstanding the terminology used by the supervisor and the supervisees to explain ethical practice. In turn, and as a consequence, it impacts on the nature of the relationship that is co-created in the process. Is this in and of itself an indication of ethical awareness?

Bacha questions whether the differences in the way each thinks about ethics are 'merely a matter of language' (Bacha, 2021: 94). Certainly, the use of language creates a problem for them both. The language used by Bacha causes Dalal to feel misunderstood and misrepresented. Perhaps Bacha feels the same and it is the use of the terms 'mutuality and reciprocity' that are key in their misunderstanding of what makes supervision ethical. Perhaps this misunderstanding provides a challenge and an opportunity for us all to think more about what is meant by these terms as evidence of ethics 'in' and 'of' supervision. Importantly I would argue that it is the co-creation of the space for dialogue and discourse, such as these exchanges demonstrate, that lifts the language of ethics off the page and brings it to life. The paucity of literature on the subject of ethics in supervision would suggest this is a long overdue concern and maybe a cause for further thought.

However, there is a caveat in this current dialogue. Both Bacha and Dalal draw on their experiences as a supervisee in a dyadic relationship with a psychoanalytic supervisor. If the concepts of mutuality and reciprocity are evidence of ethical supervisory practice in a dyad, do they easily translate to a group supervision setting?

Power and authority

The UKCP Code of Ethics and Professional Practice states, 'Be aware of the power imbalance between the practitioner and the client' (UKCP, 2019: 2).

Power is ever present as is powerlessness, but into whom do we project power and what would happen if we took back these projections and began to think more about the overarching dilemma of how we respond to change? The unique relationships co-created in the consulting room between the clinician/supervisor and the patient/supervisee contains a power dynamic. The issue of power is always present in every relationship and so will be a factor in the work we undertake in the consulting room. The question then is one of how we address it and more importantly perhaps if we acknowledge it as something to be aware of.

The dilemma for us all is how to manage both in a culture in which a power dynamic is most certainly a factor. For in the event of a complaint the spoken word of the practitioner may not hold as much weight and may be without the same level of authority as the written word of the published chapter and verse of an ethics policy. The result of this unequal relationship between our professional practice and a legalistic framework might not only be fraught with dilemmas but may add to them by omission. For example, any policy set in a time warp of unchanging social and cultural change may be out of step with the needs of the clinician in the moment.

The recent COVID-19 pandemic is just one example. In the event of this sudden departure from the usual face-to-face practice of seeing patients and supervisees in a dedicated physical space, clinicians needed to change their practices almost overnight. Virtual sessions for trainees and patients have now become the norm and guidelines and criteria have had to be hastily thought about and adapted to fit this new norm. However, where has this left the issue of ethics with reference to the virtual relationship that is co-created between clinician and patient? If there are ethical issues associated with change, as we might expect, then do we notice them or do we just turn 'a blind eye' and a 'deaf ear' hoping someone else will alert us to them, as and when necessary?

The revised Guidelines were written after the onset of the change in practice and were done so in the light of the experience of seasoned practitioners and trainees having to suddenly adapt to new ways of working. Trainees and practitioners engaged in a mutual endeavour through conversations in supervision about how best to manage the challenge of online remote sessions while maintaining an ethical framework. There is probably still a lot more work to do in this area, and we learn as we go along, but in some perverse way one might see the pandemic as an opportunity for us all to engage in a dialogue about ethical practice that will inform the legal eagles. The tables turned suddenly and, in some sense, pivoted towards the recognition of practitioner knowledge and understanding of ethical boundaries that could be called upon to influence the changes that affect us all in our relationships with patients, especially for trainees completing their training.

This experience puts us, as clinicians, in a more assertive and powerful relationship to our practice while at the same time diluting the fear of the regulatory framework. It also raises many more ethical dilemmas that are shared and creates the need to address them as a shared experience. A somewhat trivial example might be: 'Is it OK to wear pyjamas when seeing patients/supervisees online?', 'Does the wearing of pyjamas impact on the supervisee/supervisor relationship and, if so, how?', and so on. Ordinary questions that stimulate the process of thinking together about issues of ethics. This is most refreshing and welcome.

The demands of cultural change based on current experiences and/or on scientific evidence necessitate a responsibility for us as supervisors to think in terms of there being non-ethical absolutes that might involve issues of safety. As the UKCP Practice Guidelines for Supervisors (2018), states,

> Recognising that there is a normative role in supervision that includes upholding the standards of good professional practice, guiding and supporting supervisees in addressing ethical issues, balancing the needs of supervisee and client and addressing issues of safely and appropriate conduct.
>
> (UKCP, 2018: 4.4, p. 4)

I believe that, while not explicitly stating, the supervisor along with the supervisee has a level of power that goes beyond the confines of the regulatory function, 'safety and appropriate conduct' being key. And key is the co-creation of a safe supervisory framework in which the development of a shared language can be fostered, a language that can take the fear out of group supervision and out of the dangers of speaking up.

Conclusion

My intention in this chapter has been to encourage us to engage with the process of taking the fear out of the ethical regulatory framework, with a justification of our clinical work as ethical. To see ourselves as having a moral courage to confront difficult issues. I proposed that as clinicians this puts us in a much stronger position while also encouraging us to engage with addressing the impact of changing cultural norms in relation to ethics and ethical practices. My experience as chair of the UKCP ethics committee suggests that COVID has inadvertently created a platform on which there is renewed interest in building conversations around the relationship of our clinical practice to the regulatory function with regard to ethics. This way of being, the adoption of an approach that questions relationships with each other, is at the heart of ethical practice. Everything we do and say, every utterance, both verbal and non-verbal, reveals a great deal about our values and the ways in which we perceive and set about creating relationships with others. All relationships and ways of relating to each other are imbued with an ethical perspective and this is what needs our constant attention. This has always been important and is ever more so in a rapidly changing cultural environment in which we now find ourselves.

Creating the space for ordinary conversations uncovers extraordinary ideas, feelings, thoughts and views that reside in the conscious and unconscious at the individual and group level. I see exploring these conversations as an absolute. And yet the task for us as supervisors is to find a shared language of ethics in which congruence is all important. Congruence mitigates the fear of the legalistic language of guidelines and policies that serve the regulatory function in the face of evidence that suggests a level of fear exists when the language of ethics raises its head above the parapet.

I firmly believe we can, as group analytic supervisors, justify our practice as ethical on the grounds that we co-create a space for 'reflexive thought', mindful of the dangers of turning a 'blind eye' and a deaf ear. It necessitates taking a stance that accepts we work within certain regulatory and clinical boundaries and acknowledges the importance of supervision training, keeping abreast of our limitations and shortfalls as human beings living in a changing world. Constant attention to the language in the group is key.

Note

1 In this chapter I make reference to United Kingdom Council for Psychotherapy (UKCP) Policies and Guidelines, which I believe are essentially equal to those of other accrediting bodies, such as the British Association for Counselling and Psychotherapy (BACP) and the British Psychological Society (BPS).

References

Bacha CS (2021) Response to Farhad Dalal's 'The Ethics of Supervision'. *Group Analysis*, 56: 90–95.

Bacha CS (2023) Response to Farad Dalal's 'The Ethics of Supervision'. *Group Analysis*, 56 (1): 90–95.

Barnett R (2005) *Supervision, Ethical Practice and the Law.* Whurr Publishers.

Behr H and Hearst L (2005) *Group-Analytic Psychotherapy: A Meeting of Minds.* Whurr Publishers.

Casement P (1985) *On Learning from the Patient.* Routledge.

Dalal F (2021; printed 2023) The Ethics of Supervision: Reciprocity, Emergence and Prefiguration. *Group Analysis*, 56 (1): 62–80.

Dalal F (2022) Au contraire … A Reply to Claire Bacha's Response to 'The Ethics of Supervision'. *Group Analysis*, 56 (1): 96–99.

Foulkes SH (1990) *Selected Papers of S.H. Foulkes: Psychoanalysis and Group Analysis.* Karnac Books.

Griffiths F (2023) The Brexit Referendum and the Inability to Mourn: Equivalence in a Large Group. In: Hopper E (ed.), *The Tripartite Matrix in the Developing Theory and Expanding Practice of Group Analysis The Social Unconscious in Persons, Groups and Societies.* Routledge, pp. 215–221.

Hopper E (ed.) (2023) *The Tripartite Matrix in the Developing Theory and Expanding Practice of Group Analysis: The Social Unconscious in Persons, Groups and Societies.* Volume 4. Taylor & Francis.

Keats J (1817) Letter to his brothers of 21 December 1817. In: www.geocities.com/Athens/Parthenon/4942/negcap.html.

Sharpe M (ed.) (1995) *The Third Eye: Supervision of Analytic Groups.* Routledge.

Shohet R (2022) 10 minutes with Robin Shohet. *Thresholds online (BACP)*. https://www.bacp.co.uk/bacp-journals/thresholds/2022/april/10-minutes-with-robin-shohet/.

Smith M and Gallop M (2023) *Group Analytic Supervision.* Routledge.

Tubert-Oklander J (2018) The Inner Organisation of the Matrix. In: Hopper E and Weinberg H (eds), *The Social Unconscious in Persons, Groups, and Societies: The Foundation Matrix Extended and Re-configured.* Volume 3. Routledge, pp. 65–85.

UKCP (2018) *The UKCP Practice Guidelines for Supervisors.* UKCP. https://www.ipss-psychotherapy.co.uk/phdi/p1.nsf/imgpages/9308_CPJASupervisionStatement(2019).pdf/$file/CPJASupervisionStatement(2019).pdf.

UKCP (2019) *UKCP Code of Ethics and Professional Practice.* UKCP.

Chapter 15

Group Supervision, Ethics and the Influence of Culture

Margaret Smith

Introduction

After defining the term ethics, the first part of this chapter begins with some snapshots of the development of ethical writing in different cultures from the Axial Age, the period from around 800 BCE to 200 CE. This is the period of time when, in many parts of the world, there was a move away from a pastoral and nomadic life to a more settled life in cities. It focuses on some of the key figures of that time who were instrumental in the development of ethical thinking and whose teachings, along with those of their disciples, still have resonance today. It notes both some differences and also the ethical values and practices in common across diverse societies. It also notes changes in the relationship between the priesthood and the rulers of the city-states.

The second part of the chapter reflects on ethical practice today, with particular reference to the overview given by Farhad Dalal in his paper 'The Ethics of Supervision' (2021), linking the ethical debates of today with those of the Axial Age.

The final part of the chapter focuses on ethics in group supervision. It places group supervision outside the formal power structure because of the need to create a secure base for thinking and reflection. It outlines some of the cultural dilemmas faced by therapists in their conversations with their clients resulting from the challenges of cross-cultural conversations. It notes the importance of staying with the discomfort that this can elicit in these exchanges and the risk of shame driving feelings underground. It suggests that when the supervision group members are able to stay with those feelings (that is, contain the feelings and think about them), then those feelings can provide a model for the therapist who is engaged in cross-cultural dialogue.

Definition of ethics

The word ethics comes from the Greek word 'ethos' (ήθος), meaning 'character'. The ancient Greeks used the term ethos referring to the underlying

DOI: 10.4324/9781032719085-20

beliefs, the character of a community, or a nation. The ethics of a nation are influenced by its predominant religious beliefs, philosophical traditions and language along with their political and economic structure. Each of these strands influence the culture transmitted through their family, friends and school during childhood.

Ethics and culture

When he was writing about group analysis, Foulkes asserted that people's culture was deeply embedded into their personality, but that because it seems 'natural' it is largely unconscious. He attributed this to the social conditioning each of us receives in childhood. He understood this conditioning to be necessary in order for us to fit into the society that we are a part of (Foulkes, 1990: 166). Conditioning takes place in the family, and tensions in the family often arise because of the norms that are accepted practice within the surrounding culture (Foulkes 1964: 141). Weinberg suggests 'Every culture ... is strongly connected to moral views' that they may be unaware of (Weinberg, 2003: 255).

Following Foulkes and Weinberg, this chapter assumes that the ethical perspectives underlying behaviour in all countries are socially conditioned and largely unconscious. They can be brought into the forefront of a person's mind by a conversation that is dissonant with their unconscious assumptions or a situation that challenges their way of behaving. This is more likely to happen in conversations with people from different backgrounds. Some of the social tensions of today surrounding gay and trans rights and culture wars can emerge in conversations in groups, and a clash of perspectives is something that can also emerge in a therapy group. In a multicultural society, or when a supervisor in one country is giving or receiving supervision in a group that is based in a different culture, there will be differences in ethical perspectives that need to be understood and thought about. With these in mind, this chapter explores the emergence of some of the world's predominant philosophies and ethics.

Foulkes' review of *The Civilizing Process* by Norbert Elias (1982) explains that:

> What is considered as 'civilized' behaviour is, however, subject to constant development. Its standards are by no means absolute but change from one country to another and from one period to another in the same country. This standard is always set by the ruling class in each society and shows a similar curve of development in the Western European countries.
>
> (Foulkes, 1990: 60)

This chapter on ethics and culture sets ethics in a historical and international political and economic context in order to understand the way they have emerged and the purpose they serve. The roots of some of the ancient thinkers who have produced work on ethical practice that has survived to this day emerged from a historical, cultural, political and economic context. Thinkers and prophets such as Socrates, Plato, Aristotle, the Buddha, Confucius, Yājñavalkya and the Old Testament prophets lived between 800 BCE to 200 CE. This was a time when society was becoming more complex and relationships extended more widely than being mainly based on kinship.

Jared Diamond argues that the precondition for changes such as these is for societies to have an agricultural system that can provide a plentiful supply of food to support larger populations in order to release some people from working on the land. This is necessary in order to support the division of labour and allow for specialisation. Having time to study and write was only possible under these circumstances. Diamond also argues that once this was established, it was an advantage because it accelerated economic growth (Diamond, 1998). In the period under consideration between 800 BCE and 200 CE, scholarship and writing flourished. Although much of the world's writing from this period has been destroyed by flood, fire or invading armies, including works from the writers mentioned below, we still have enough to piece together some of the texts on ethics, morals and etiquette.

Karl Jaspers coined the term 'the Axial Age', to encompass this period, tracing the emerging religious and philosophical thought that took place at this time (Jaspers, 1948). Although there is some disagreement among scholars about the usefulness of defining the Axial Age as a distinct period, this chapter uses it because it provides a useful lens through which to look at the developments taking place during this period. David Graeber points out that it was during the period of the Axial Age that a number of the world's great religions were established: Zoroastrianism, Prophetic Judaism, Buddhism, Jainism, Hinduism, Confucianism, Taoism, Christianity and Hellenism (following the gods of ancient Greece). Some of the great ethical thinkers, Buddha, Confucius, Pythagoras, Aristotle and Plato also date back to this period. It was in some of these areas that coinage first arose, for example in India, China and Judaea. Graeber attributes this to the ethical codes embedded in the religious beliefs of these cultures. This was only possible because of the moral standards that there was the trust needed to use money in exchanges between people who did not know each other (Graeber, 2009).

Part 1: The Axial Age and the rise of religion, philosophy and ethics

This section focuses on the emergence and ethical practices of Eastern perspectives connected with their respective religious traditions. It connects them with some of the social, political and economic factors that underpin them to contextualise their formation.

The teachings about ethics from the Axial Age were woven into the religious beliefs of the day. Many of the ethical principles contained in the writings of the major religions from this period are similar. What is different is often the motivation behind their use. For the writers from Judaism and Christianity, keeping the ten commandments and loving your neighbour as yourself (Mark 12: 30–31) are a part of living in a right relationship with God. They are principles that are demanded by God, who will judge and punish sin. For Buddhists and Hindus, living a good life offers hope that one day they will attain enlightenment and escape from the cycle of birth and rebirth. For Confucians, life is inevitably about suffering. It is possible to learn from suffering and to learn how to live a virtuous life in order to escape the cycle of birth and death. In Hinduism, there is a belief in divine punishment and that individuals will live with the consequences of their behaviour both in this life or and in future reincarnations.

The emergence of ethical thinking during the Axial Age

The move from a pastoral life based in clans, to one where people were closely connected, to one where people lived in cities with others who were strangers was the defining shift of the period. In the city-states, everyone was either connected with the ruling class or was one of their subjects. There was often a gulf between the wealthy elites and the majority of people, who were poor. Goods were no longer shared and some people had control over others. From the perspective of the state, social harmony was vital for the rulers to keep a hold of their power and the threat of their subjects receiving divine punishment for rebellious behaviour, now or in times to come served them well. It also helped to maintain the inequalities of wealth that were endemic during this period. This was a disadvantage for the poor and needy, who suffered the consequences of their deprivations.

Merlin Donald argues that in these more complex societies of the Axial Age, it was the religious beliefs and practices that supported societal cohesion. Each society followed the same pattern, although these patterns took different forms. These forms included the 'regulatory structures ... that were enshrined in the beliefs and practices and embedded through their religious rituals. These rituals required people to monitor and evaluate their behavior and to make changes when they did not fit in with their society's norms' (Donald, 2012: 73).

The religious founders were surrounded by myth: most came from privileged or wealthy backgrounds, often being princes or noblemen; the founders of these religious traditions were teachers who had disciples who recorded their teachings; they founded religious traditions that enshrined ethical principles linked to the worship of God or the gods. They were seen as outsiders—Bellah refers to them as 'the renouncers', people who spoke against the rulers of the day. They were often persecuted for their teachings, and some were sentenced to death (Bellah and Joas, 2012: 451). Each of these is explored in more detail.

1. Founders of world religions that arose during this period

The Axial Age was one where writing was still limited to a small percentage of the population. Some of the great thinkers and prophets, who are now surrounded by myth, had disciples and scribes recording their sayings. By using 'form criticism' (analysing the style of writing) and redaction criticism (looking at editorial content), we know from the work of scholars that the writings of these thinkers and prophets were compiled and sometimes added to. Much of what we know about the founders of these religions was written down after their deaths by their disciples, sometimes generations after they had died. Myths survive over time because of the truths contained within them that speak to people across the generations. What is important for the purposes of this chapter is not the historical accuracy of the accounts but rather the emerging picture that has shaped the nature of our ethical thinking over the centuries.

2. Religious founders of noble or royal birth and privileged backgrounds

Confucius's early ancestors were the Kongs from the state of Song. He was from an aristocratic family where several of his forebears were eminent advisors to the Song rulers. We know one of his writings, *The Book of Documents*, contained speeches by emperors and politicians (Peng et al., 2024). This suggests a connection with the rulers of the day. One of the best-known Hindu Vedic sages was Yājñavalkya. He was believed to have been born into a Brahmin family and given a good education. He went on to become a scholar showing a deep commitment to gain knowledge and the pursuit of wisdom, something highly valued at that time. The Buddha was a noble prince who renounced his wealth and lived as a monk, in spite of pressure from family and one of the local kings to return.

The lineage of the prophets of the Old Testament was mentioned where known and they crossed paths with the priests and rulers of the day. The Book of Elijah connects the prophet Elijah with King Ahab who had Naboth, a local farmer, murdered in order to steal his vineyard at the request of Queen Jezebel. Elijah confronted Ahab who repented, but Elijah was forced to escape from Queen Jezebel's wrath (1 Kings 21: 20–28). The prophet Jeremiah had a priestly lineage and had dealings with King Jehoiakim (Jeremiah 36: 1–32). Christ was of royal descent (Luke 2: 4). Tim Gee, who studied the accounts of Christ's life, has proposed that the accounts in the gospels can be read to suggest that Christ was seen as a revolutionary and in direct conflict with the Roman occupying forces (Gee, 2022).

3. Founders as outsiders

It was during this time that relationships changed between the state, supported by the military, and the priesthood. Initially state and priesthood were separate but interconnected. However, over time, the two became distinct from each other (Eisenstadt, 2012: 280). Each of these traditions contained ethical teachings that challenged the rulers as well as their subjects to live a good life. Obeyesekere points out that the Buddha's decision to leave was as a result of the corruption of court life. 'Once the Buddha decided to become a renouncer, he ceased to be a member of the local community' (Obeyesekere, 2012: 140). While it is true that most of the world's religious founders were from privileged backgrounds, their ethical teachings placed them as outsiders within their societies. From their positions as outsiders (Buddha, Confucius, the Old Testament prophets, Christ, Aristotle and Plato) were prepared to speak out about the corruption and injustices of the day (Assman 2012; Bellah and Joas 2012; Martin 2012; Obeyesekere, 2012; Runciman 2012).

Common to all was their devotion to living out the spiritual life demanded by their faith regardless of the consequences. This was certainly true of the Buddha, who lived as an outcast. And the Upanishads suggests that Yājña-valkya was a Hindu sage who did not conform to the norms of his day. The prophets of the Torah were all outsiders, devoting their lives to speaking truth to power (that is, speaking out against injustice and corruption to the people who were in positions of power) and urging people to return to God. This was also true of Christ, who is recorded as spending time in the Temple as he was growing up, but who challenged both the religious leaders and the Roman rulers of his day.

4. Some founders were persecuted or sentenced to death

The role of the outsider was to hold a mirror to what was happening within their society and to name the injustice and corruption within it. This is not without risk. The consequences of speaking truth to power were persecution and death. Jeremiah was thrown into a cistern (a deep hole in the ground), in this case one with mud at the bottom, which Jeremiah was stuck in (Jeremiah 38: 6). Socrates and Christ were condemned to death. Each is shown to have chosen their role. The prophets were able to speak out because of their unshakeable belief that they were speaking the word of God and that they would be vindicated. As Job, another of the prophets, said when faced with derision 'I know that my redeemer lives, and that in the end he will stand on the earth. And after my skin has been destroyed, yet in my flesh I will see God; I myself will see him with my own eyes (Job 19: 25–27). Socrates is understood to have taught his disciples, but he spoke out publicly only at the end of his life. He was unpopular for questioning the teachings of the elders, and because of his 'impropriety' in not following the gods that were supported by the state. Plato records that the death of Socrates followed a trial brought against him for this and that he chose to die in prison by suicide. Christ was crucified because he spoke out about the corruption in the Temple at Jerusalem and he was said by some to have claimed to be the king of the Jews.

Summary of the ethical teachings of the Axial Age

The world's religions are each shaped according to the cultures where they arose and the personalities of the founders, as conveyed in the writings of their disciples. This also applies to the ethics contained within their messages.

For Confucianism, writings about religion and ethics are intertwined. It is founded on 'ren', compassion and care for others, which was the highest moral principle. Other virtues included respect and social harmony, filial piety, loyalty and honesty. These five virtues begin with the individual, but encompass societies and nations. These would have been useful to the ruling classes, too, because they give guidance about how to maintain social harmony and the proper ordering of society. The four noble truths that are the foundation of Buddhism are: (1) *Dukkha*, the realisation of suffering; (2) *Samudaya*, an understanding that suffering arises through craving; (3) *Nirodha*, the hope that comes from believing that suffering will end; and (4) *Magga*, the belief that there is a path that can lead to the cessation of suffering. The purpose of the four noble truths is to link suffering in the world with people's greed. It teaches how to free ourselves from the addictions that drive our greed by living according to the eightfold path. This required ethical living, meditation and developing wisdom. The eightfold path has been summarised as 'Right View, Right Intention, Right Speech, Right Action, Right Livelihood, Right Effort, Right Mindfulness, and Right Concentration' (Ta, 2025).

Hindu ethics are closely related to Buddhism. Both stress the importance of Dharma. Hinduism includes the virtues of compassion, truthfulness, and righteousness. In Hinduism, dharma the religious and moral law governs individual conduct that is one of the four ends of life. The ethics of Judaism unfold over the course of the Torah. The prophet Moses is said to have received the ten commandments directly from God and the five that encompass societal living include

> … you shall not murder, you shall not commit adultery. You shall not steal, you shall not give false testimony against your neighbour and you shall not covet your neighbour's house. You shall not covet your neighbour's wife, or his male or female servant, his ox or donkey, or anything that belongs to your neighbour.
>
> (Exodus 20: 13–20)

The prophets preached against the rulers and people who turned away from the true religion. Hosea sees this turning away from God as intertwined with the corruption of Israelite society. 'There is no truth, no loving devotion, and no knowledge of God in the land! Cursing and lying, murder and stealing, and adultery are rampant; one act of bloodshed follows another' (Hosea 4: 1–2).

Christ's ethical teachings are found in the 'Sermon on the Mount'. Matthew's account stresses the virtues of the spiritual life (Matthew: 5–7). Luke's version promises a place in the kingdom of God the poor, comfort for those who weep, and blessings and the promise of Heaven to those who suffer in his name. He condemns the rich and asks the crowd to love and pray for their enemies and to turn the other cheek when struck. They should give without expecting anything in return. They should be merciful, as God is, and, rather than judging others, they should examine their own lives for shortcomings (Luke 6: 20–42).

The ethical teachings of the Axial Age: religious and societal perspectives

Many of the ethical principles contained in the writings of the major religions from this period are similar. What is different is the motivation behind right living. For the writers from Judaism and Christianity, keeping the ten commandments and loving your neighbour as yourself (Mark 12: 30–31) are a part of living in a right relationship with God. They are principles demanded by God who will judge and punish sin. For Buddhists and Hindus, living a good life offers hope that one day they will attain enlightenment and escape from the cycle of birth and rebirth. For Confucians, life is inevitably about suffering. It is possible to learn from suffering how to live a virtuous life in order to escape the cycle of birth and death. In Hinduism, there is a belief in the divine and that individuals will live with the consequences of their behaviour both in this life and/or in future reincarnations.

The religious teachings from the Axial Age also supported the maintenance of social order and the law within society. For example, the ten commandments may have influenced the laws of many countries today. The greed of one person affects the wealth of others around them and having a religious tradition that created the stricture that this would affect their ability to reach enlightenment was a way of regulating behaviour. Compassion, being kind to others, can help people to relate to others they do not know and avoid hurting them. Societal living is made easier when there is trust. It is fundamental to our lives. Trust is needed in our day-to-day lives and this includes the monetary exchanges made with the people who supply our food, clothing and shelter. Trust is only possible when someone is honest and truthful. Loyalty is something needed not just in the family but also at the state level. For example, serving in the military requires loyalty to the state. These teachings were underpinned by the moral code with sanctions for breaches from a higher power in this life and the next.

This examination of the development of ethical thinking during the Axial Age has limitations. For example, it does not include the development of ethical thinking and practice from early societies on the continents of Africa and America. For example, there were city states such as Copán Tikal, and Palenque, with rulers and priests who recorded their texts in Mayan society. Likewise in Africa, city states included Cairo and Alexandria in Egypt, Carthage in Modern day Tunisia, Axum in Ethiopia. Study of these may provide further insight into the history of ethical development as it emerged in these places.

Part 2: The Axial Age as the root of our ethical debates today

In the recent paper by Farhad Dalal about ethics and supervision, Dalal divides ethics into three strands. First, deontology, the Greek term for duty. In the deontological model, ethics originated using rational argument to deduce the correct way to live. Once arrived at, they become rules that should be followed regardless of consequences. He gives the example that duty requires a person to always tell the truth in each and every circumstance, even if an innocent person will be injured by the consequences (Dalal, 2021: 8).

Second, Dalal mentions consequentialism. This is a term that covers both hedonism, the imperative to maximise pleasure, with its roots going back to ancient Greece, and utilitarianism, the imperative to create the greatest good for the greatest number (Dalal, 2021: 8).

Third, Dalal describes virtue ethics. According to Aristotle, virtue ethics are things we learn as we assimilate the culture around us during childhood. These then become the habits that inform our actions. Dalal points out virtue ethics are about how we feel rather than how we are thinking. His contention is that, because ethics have been internalised, they are not just cognitive rules but also elicit an emotional response. When there is what he calls 'ethical distress', where something just does not feel right to someone, this is responding at an emotional level. This type of response to an ethical dilemma, Dalal suggests, requires a different language. He quotes Pascal's well-known saying 'The Heart has its reasons that Reason cannot understand' (Dalal, 2021).

Each of these three perspectives on ethics, each approaching the subject from a different perspective, can be traced to speeches given by religious thinkers from the age of classical Greece. There are some debates about whether in Plato's portrayal of Socrates took a deductive deontological approach or whether he applied virtue ethics (Ohtani, 2022). Creed wrote a paper called 'Is it Wrong to Call Plato A Utilitarian?' (Creed, 1978). The overall message here is that the questions that preoccupied the ancient Greeks contained the seeds of our ethical debates in Western cultures today.

We have seen that the ethics of Buddhism, Hinduism, Confucianism, Judaism and Christianity have roots in different cultural traditions. These traditions too continue to influence some of the different and rich perspectives that are reflected in our increasingly multicultural society.

Part 3: Ethics and the culture of group supervision

Group supervision is space that allows for thinking and reflection about therapeutic relationships. Members are aware of formal channels of power within their workplace, but supervision stands outside of this. In order to practise, they need to belong to a professional body and adhere to the codes of ethics drawn up by their organisation. Codes of ethics often read rather like the ten commandments—examples of deontological ethics where a code of conduct is presented to people who must follow them or face sanctions. Within the context of supervision, the task is to focus on the things that the therapist finds difficult to navigate in their work. There can be a tension between being completely open and hiding things felt to be shaming—for example, the tension between being completely open about feelings, attitudes and responses or hiding them in order not to be seen as wanting. It may never be known how far the fear of judgement, as a result of a therapist revealing something they feel uncomfortable about in front of their supervisor and their peers, may limit what is said. While there are examples of these codes of ethics being violated, this is not the main focus in a chapter on group supervision and the influence of culture.

If we take seriously what Foulkes said about all of us being 'pre-conditioned to the core by his community, even before he is born, and his personality and character are imprinted vitally by the group in which he is raised' (Foulkes, 1990: 152), we need to acknowledge that none of us are neutral players. In group supervision, we come with our own cultural bias and this needs to be taken into account when thinking about the work under discussion.

When a dilemma arises in group supervision that involves a clash of culture this can be a challenge for us. Most of the time we may not be conscious of our moral biases, but we all have them. This is the part of us that Foulkes refers to as the 'so-called inner processes in the individual ... internalisations of the forces operating in the group to which he belongs' (Foulkes, 1990: 212). At times when cultural perspectives differ, either in the work of the therapy or in the supervision group, it is important to find a way to talk about it. Nollaig Byrne coined the phrase 'diamond absolutes' to describe the impossibility of a mother from a Protestant culture discussing her abortion with her Catholic daughter (Byrne, 1995). They have each internalised messages containing the social mores from these respective cultures (Foulkes, 1990: 212). Under circumstances such as these, it may be easy to get diverted into enacting the parallel process that, in the case of this example, was the harsh judgement of the daughter. Or a supervision group may get drawn into taking the opposite stance and identifying with the position of the mother. To begin a conversation that steers between these two involves the capacity to stand back and see the bigger picture. The task is not to cast judgement, but rather to try to understand the process. I have seen this done in a family session when a family was seemingly at war, and the therapist was unsure how to proceed. Members of the observing group were asked to speak for each of the people in the family therapy session, each speaking for a different family member. This allowed members of the observing group to take ownership of their positions and it was useful learning for them. It also allowed for all voices to be represented, including some from the family group who had been silent in the session. It may have been the capacity of the supervision group members to tune in at an emotional level (virtue ethics) that allowed the group to think about the family as a whole, introducing different perspectives that then freed up communication with the family in the subsequent session.

Another dilemma occurs when there is a difference in the culture of the supervision group itself. For example, when a therapist from India is in a mixed Zoom supervision group and is the only person from that country. When they present their client, they bring someone who is depressed because of the strictures of family life. Their father is perceived as domineering and their mother as submissive. They are trapped because, although they are an adult, they do not earn enough money to leave home. According to a report by the British Neuropathological Society (BNS) Institute entitled 'Analyzing the Status and Roles of Women in Indian Families', women in Indian society have experienced inequality with men and this has been shown to reduce their overall quality of life. Although this is changing, their status in society, the responsibility they carry within the home, and their resultant dependence on men for financial support, leave them with less power (BNS Institute, 2023. As Foulkes reminds us, 'illness is interpersonal and involves the community' (Foulkes, 1964: 296). When I was faced with a similar situation a few years ago, I had the experience described by Dalal that there was something that did not feel right about proceeding as though the work we were discussing was located in the West. It would be easy for a White woman to get caught up in thinking about the limitations placed on this woman as equivalent in some way to the experiences of women in the West. The two situations may be similar, but they are not equivalent as women in the West enjoy greater autonomy. It is important for the supervision group to draw on empathy based on their own experience while also staying curious about how it may be different for someone from another cultural tradition.

As well as the issue of differences in culture, there is the issue of race. This is complicated by not just being about differences in cultural norms and histories. This is about people who may have a family history of being systematically uprooted and enslaved for the enrichment of one race at the expense of another. The trauma resulting from this can often be alive, generations after the events that took place. There can be an additional discomfort in speaking about race and its legacy that can be very hard to acknowledge. Reem Shelhi movingly explores this in her chapter called 'This Is How I Came to Live in Stuckness',

Taking a group analytic setting as a microcosm of the larger cultural-socio-political environment, I draw on post-colonial and Black Feminist literature along with my experience of training as a group analyst, to magnify how different axes of oppression can interlock, forming sedimented intersectional knots of stuckness and immobility that, if overlooked, ignored or denied, find explosive expression in affects which the social realm condemns as unwelcome disturbances (Fanon, 2018). I argue that turning away from these affects maintains a climate of socio-intersectional anxiety and alienation, precipitating further disturbances and perpetuating cycles of rage and despair. I propose an intervention I term 'Affectivism' as a means of amplifying silenced voices and 'calling out' oppressive situations.

(Shelhi, 2024: 194–195)

The challenge this poses is not an easy one to overcome and cannot be initiated without commitment to face this head on. In his book, *The Race Conversation*, Eugene Ellis reminds us that it is not possible to truly engage in a conversation about race without it bringing discomfort. This may be avoided or brushed over because it feels too difficult and it may lead to rationalisation. It requires a willing commitment to embrace the discomfort to begin the journey. Ellis refers to the difficulties that are faced when engaging in such conversations as 'the race construct'. This, he suggests is 'a way of splitting self and other that serves to alleviate any internal discomfort in white people' (Ellis, 2021: 91).

Shelhi generously describes the damage she experiences as someone from an ethnic minority living in this country. This is as a result of feeling on the outside but needing a way of relating to people that allows some limited connection, though without the emotional shielding available to those living on the inside. This comes at a significant personal cost. She says:

We orbit around ourselves from a distance that paradoxically keeps us connected in ways that don't threaten to split and fragment us into ever tinier pieces. From this outpost, we see the bigger picture clearly. At the same time, perhaps because taken-for-granted truths are not so readily available to us, we insist on the truth wherever we find it. As Cone says, 'a helpful duping of oneself to soften the blow is not available'.

(Shelhi, 2024)

This poignant description invites us to engage in a more genuine and constructive way in spite of our discomfort. In *The Race Conversation*, Ellis (2021: 79–81) outlines the five aspects of the race construct. They are: situation-specific shame; physiological responses to shame; the infectious nature of shame; the unravelling of our identity; and managing their critical inner voice. It begins with shame being triggered. The shame has been remembered and passed from one generation to the next 'non-verbally and in implicit ways'. The experience of shame affects the body of the people affected creating a sensation of disintegration and isolation. These feelings of shame can affect everyone involved. They are infectious and dysregulating because they occur between people who do not respond with the emotional connection needed to help them regain their emotional balance. This is because the people in the conversation are likely to pick up danger signals, affecting them bodily and this too is infectious. This can lead to what Ellis calls an experience of unravelling, where a person begins to question their identity, with such questions as are we a good person, or are we a racist? They may feel that their identity is 'being held up for inspection and found wanting'. This can lead to a person trying to protect the wound they are experiencing by either trying too hard to prove themselves or by getting in touch with simmering anger (Shelhi, 2024: 224).

Shelhi warns us that:

> Oppressive conduct couched in clinical interventions is easy to detect by the receiver but often difficult to substantiate, particularly when oppressions intersect and overlap, making distinctions between them seem impossible. As clinicians, this places us in positions of responsibility while accentuating the importance of honesty and integrity in our conduct.
>
> (Shelhi, 2024: 216)

Shelhi is highlighting one of the problems inherent in asymmetric relationships, such as that between the therapist and their group members. She reminds the reader not to abuse the power invested in conductors and of the importance of mental hygiene (Shelhi, 2024: 216). Group supervision is an ideal place for this mental hygiene to take place through self-examination in the supervision group where they take their work.

Ellis invites therapists to, 'go beyond a shallow understanding of race and keep connected with what is important' but recognises that

> we will need a strategy to manage discomfort. In my experience of working with race trauma, what seems to be most important is to keep connected to the hurt that race inflicts on people of colour predominately but also white people. I am referring to hurt transmitted over generations which continues to be inflicted in the present. It is this focus within the race conversation that I believe will bring about healing and change.
>
> (Ellis, 2021: 20–21)

The supervision group sits outside of the work that the therapist is engaged with. In a well-functioning group, this can make it easier to sit with the discomfort that is brought into the room when a therapist talks openly about their feelings when they bring their emotional response to the trauma affecting people experiencing racism. The task of the supervision group is to stay with the discomfort, acting as a container for the pain, while being open about the way the material resonates for them emotionally and physically. Where a supervision group is drawn from people from different cultures, this may help them all to see that there is no comfortable position, whether they are experiencing themselves as victims, perpetrators or bystanders. I suggest that when the supervision group are able to stay with the feelings and talk about them openly this can provide a model for the therapist who is engaged in cross-cultural dialogue about the trauma of racism in their therapy group.

Conclusion

The ethical perspectives that are debated today have their roots in the Axial Age that occurred during the thousand years between around 800 BCE and 200 CE in city-states. This is where some of the families who could afford to educate their children had sufficient wealth for the families to support them in becoming teachers and priests. The founders of the major religions (Socrates, Plato, Aristotle, the Buddha, Confucius, Yājñavalkya, Christ and the Old Testament prophets of this period) were both well connected and seen as outsiders. From them we have the ethical developments contained within the works of Confucius, the Upanishads (containing the work of Yājñavalkya), the Bible and the writings of the Buddha. Over time, there was a separation between the priesthood and the state. From the position of outsiders, they condemned the corruption of the state and the lack of religious piety and spoke out about the injustices of the day. Their wisdom and the ethical debates they engaged in were recorded by their disciples and became the sacred texts we know today.

When working with ethical dilemmas that relate to differences in cultural perspectives, group supervision, with its capacity to step back a little, can help in seeing the bigger picture. When the members of the supervision group are able to engage in conversations about the emotional content of the work and its impact on them, this can aid the therapist in staying with discomfort. It does this by providing a model they can carry with them back into the therapy room.

References

Assman J (2012) Cultural Memory and the Myth of the Axial Age. In: Bellah RN and Joas H (eds), *The Axial Age and Its Consequences*. Harvard University Press.

Bellah RN and Joas H (eds) (2012). *The Axial Age and Its Consequences*. Harvard University Press.

Bible, The. (2011) New International Version. HarperCollins Christian Publishing.

BNS Institute (2023). Analyzing the Status and Roles of Women in Indian Families. Available at https://bns.institute/behavioural-sciences/status-roles-women-indian-families/.

Byrne N (1995) A Daughter's Response to her Mother's Abortion. *Human Systems: The Journal of Systemic Consultation and Management*, 6: 255–277.

Creed JL (1978) Is it Wrong to Call Plato A Utilitarian? *The Classical Quarterly*, 28 (2): 349–365.

Dalal F (2021) The Ethics of Supervision: Reciprocity, Emergence and Prefiguration. *Group Analysis*, 56: 62–80.

Diamond J (1998) *Guns, Germs and Steel*. Vintage.

Donald M (2012) An Evolutionary Approach to Culture: Implications for the Study of the Axial Age. In: Bellah RN and Joas H (eds), *The Axial Age and Its Consequences*. Harvard University Press.

Elias N (1982). *The Civilizing Process: State Formation and Civilization*, translated by Edmund Jephcott (with notes and revisions by the author). Blackwell.

Ellis E (2021) *The Race Conversation: An Essential Guide to Creating Life-Changing Dialogue*. Confer Books.

Exodus (2011) *The Bible*. New International Version. HarperCollins Christian Publishing.

Fanon F (2018 [2021]). *Black Skin, White Masks*. Paladin.

Foulkes SH (1964) *Therapeutic Group Analysis*. George Allen and Unwin.

Foulkes SH (1990) *Selected Papers of S.H. Foulkes: Psychoanalysis and Group Analysis*. Karnac Books.

Gee T (2022) *Open for Liberation. An Activist Reads the Bible*. Christian Alternative Books.

Graeber D (2009) *Debt: The First Five Thousand Years*. Melville House Publishing

Hosea (2011) *The Bible*. New International Version. HarperCollins Christian Publishing.

Jaspers K (1948). *Der philosophische Glaube angesichts der Offenbarung*. Artemis.

Jeremiah (2011) *The Bible*. New International Version. HarperCollins Christian Publishing.

Job (2011) *The Bible*. New International Version. HarperCollins Christian Publishing.

Kings (1) (2011) *The Bible*. New International Version. HarperCollins Christian Publishing.

Luke (2011) *The Bible*. New International Version. HarperCollins Christian Publishing.

Mark (2011) *The Bible*. New International Version. HarperCollins Christian Publishing.

Martin D (2012) Axial Religions and the Problem of Violence. In: Bellah RN and Joas H (eds), *The Axial Age and Its Consequences*. Harvard University Press, pp. 294–316.

Matthew (2011) *The Bible*. New International Version. HarperCollins Christian Publishing.

Obeyesekere G (2012) The Buddha's Meditative Trance: Visionary Knowledge, Aphoristic Thinking, and Axial Age Rationality in Early Buddhism. In: Bellah RN and Joas H (eds), *The Axial Age and Its Consequences*. Harvard University Press, pp. 126–145.

Ohtani H (2022) Personal and Objective Ethics: How to Read the Crito. *Philosophy*, 97(1): 91–114.

Peng P (2025). Meritocracy Reimagined: Ideational Foundations of State-Building in Imperial China. *Journal of Historical Political Economy*, 4(4), 439–469.

Runciman WG (2012) Righteous Rebels: When, Where and Why. In: Bellah RN and Joas H (eds), *The Axial Age and Its Consequences*. Harvard University Press.

Shelhi R (2024) This Is How I Came to Live in Stuckness. In: Nayak S and Forrest A (eds), *Intersectionality and Group Analysis: Explorations of Power, Privilege, and Position in Group Therapy.* Taylor & Francis.

Ta D (2025) The Buddha Student. https://buddhastudent.com/.

Weinberg H (2003) The Culture of the Group and Groups from Different Cultures. *Group Analysis,* 36: 253–268.

Index

For Product Safety Concerns and Information please contact our EU
representative GPSR@taylorandfrancis.com
Taylor & Francis Verlag GmbH, Kaufingerstraße 24, 80331 München, Germany

9 781032 719054